WADE HAMPTON FROST,
PIONEER EPIDEMIOLOGIST 1880–1938

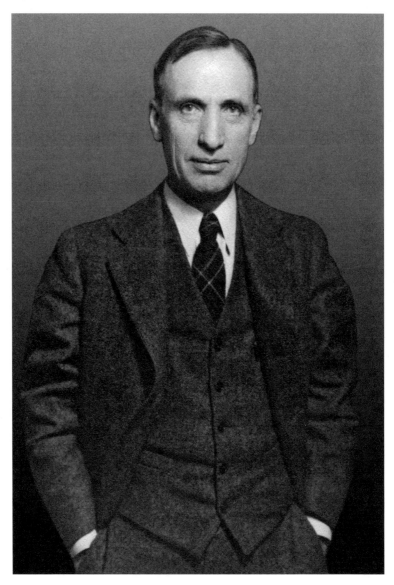

Wade Hampton Frost. This portrait was painted by Julia Godine working from photographs of Frost in 1988 on commission from Jack M. Gwaltney Jr., Wade Hampton Frost Professor of Medicine at the University of Virginia. It now hangs in the Epidemiology Conference Room, Cobb Hall, University of Virginia Medical Center. Reproduced from a photograph, with permission courtesy of the Historical Collection and Services in the Claude Moore Health Sciences Library, University of Virginia Health Sciences Center, Charlottesville, Va.: Wade Hampton Frost Archives.

WADE HAMPTON FROST, PIONEER EPIDEMIOLOGIST 1880–1938

Up to the Mountain

Thomas M. Daniel

University of Rochester Press

First published 2004

University of Rochester Press
668 Mount Hope Avenue
Rochester, NY 14620 USA
www.urpress.com

and at Boydell & Brewer, Ltd.
P.O. Box 9
Woodbridge, Suffolk IP12 3DF
www.boydellandbrewer.com

ISBN 1–58046–177–8

Library of Congress Cataloging-in-Publication Data

Daniel, Thomas M.
  Wade Hampton Frost, pioneer epidemiologist 1880–1938 : Up to the mountain /
Thomas M. Daniel.
     p. ; cm.
  Includes bibliographical references and index.
  ISBN 1–58046–177–8 (hardcover : alk. paper)
  1. Frost, Wade Hampton, 1880–1938.   2. Epidemiologists—United
States—Biography.   I. Title.
  [DNLM: 1. Frost, Wade Hampton, 1880–1938.   2. Epidemiology—Biography.   3.
Physicians—Biography. WZ 100 D1844u 2004]
  RA649.5.F76D366 2004
  614.4′092–dc22
  [B]

                                                              2004013877

British Library Cataloguing-in-Publication Data
A catalogue record for this book
is available from the British Library.

Printed in the USA.
This publication is printed on Acid Free Paper.

Come ye, and let us go up to the mountain, . . .
and he will teach us of his ways, and we
will walk in his path.

Isaiah 2:3

Contents

Figures

Tables

Foreword

Throughout my career in epidemiology, which has spanned much of the twentieth century, I often heard references to Wade Hampton Frost as the one who did the most to bring epidemiology into the ranks of scientific disciplines. And yet, when I recently looked through the medley of epidemiology textbooks in my library, I found his name mentioned in only about half of them, and then usually in connection with his paper on cohort analysis.[1] There was one notable exception. John R. Paul, in his book, *Clinical Epidemiology*, said:

> Frost did much to transform epidemiology in the United States from a loose discipline to an analytical and productive science. Frost's work began with careful clinical observations, many of which were made as part of a series of field observations; this was followed up with population measurements. Then with orderly precision the data were subjected to biostatistical treatment. It had taken almost four thousand years for epidemiology to emerge as a discipline ready, by about 1920, to stand on its own feet among the medical arts and sciences. To Frost also we owe in part the concept that an epidemic is but a temporary phase in the occurrence of any disease and as such epidemiology represented more than the study of epidemics and was a science ready to be applied to all diseases.[2]

Few would disagree with Paul's assessment of Frost's work, a fact that makes the scant attention paid to Frost by the teachers of epidemiology in their textbooks puzzling. It cannot be that his name was forgotten; half of the texts did refer to one of his papers. Furthermore, in 1972 the Epidemiology Section of the American Public Health Association initiated a series of Wade Hampton Frost lectures at its annual meetings; these were continued for more than two decades, although, unfortunately, relatively few were published.

Several of the earlier lectures emphasized the different facets of epidemiology to which Frost had contributed. In the first lecture, Abraham Lilienfeld reviewed the progressive spread of epidemiologic methods to the study of chronic noninfectious diseases, a trend started by Frost.[3] John Fox noted Frost's pioneering use of the family as a unit for epidemiologic study.[4] John Cassell started with Frost's statement:

> Epidemiology at any given time is something more than the total of its established facts. It includes their orderly arrangement into chains of inference which extend beyond the bounds of direct observation.[5]

Cassel then constructed his own orderly arrangement of facts, producing a convincing argument that social environment could affect host resistance. Somewhat later, Milton Terris made a plea to his colleagues and successors to follow Frost's example by continuing the epidemiologic tradition of applying research findings to the improvement of the public's health.[6] Terris closed his lecture by saying that Frost and many other epidemiologists would approve Horace Mann's sentiments. In his final address to the graduates of Antioch College, Mann concluded:

> I beseech you to treasure up in your hearts these my parting words. Be ashamed to die until you have won some victory for humanity![7]

When several senior epidemiologists find such breadth of wisdom in Frost's epidemiologic thinking, it is surpassing strange that modern teachers mention his works so infrequently. Is it disdain for the simpler nature of epidemiology in the past with its lack of significance tests and complex mathematical analysis? Is it ignorance of preelectronic citations? Or is it that so much of Frost's teaching became manifest primarily through the work of his students?[8] Whatever the reason, Frost, the man, the teacher, and the epidemiologist *par excellence* deserves to be better known today. Tom Daniel has produced a scholarly and entertaining story of the life and works of Wade Hampton Frost. It will interest and instruct a broad spectrum of readers both in and outside the field of medicine.

GEORGE W. COMSTOCK, M.D., DR.P.H., F.A.C.E.

Alumni Centennial Professor
Emeritus of Epidemiology
Johns Hopkins University Bloomberg
School of Public Health

Preface

I first became aware of the work of Wade Hampton Frost many years ago when, as a young faculty member, I was given the responsibility of organizing and presenting much of the curricular material on tuberculosis for medical students at my university. I was not then and am not now an epidemiologist, but it was apparent to me that my teaching would have to include the epidemiology of tuberculosis. My knowledge of the clinical disease was not enough. I began reading and studying. It became clear to me that I would have to present Frost's cohort analyses of the age selection of tuberculosis mortality. Without this major work, one could not understand the age-specific case rates for tuberculosis in the United States and elsewhere in the world.

Many years later I moved to emeritus status at Case Western Reserve University, and I began writing medical history. By this time, I had a greater appreciation of Frost's importance, and I decided to include him in a book profiling six great medical pioneers (*Pioneers of Medicine and Their Impact on Tuberculosis*, University of Rochester Press, 2000). In the process I discovered, first, that no biography of Frost had been written, although a number of short biographical sketches had appeared, and, second, that all of Frost's personal papers had been archived at the University of Virginia. It was apparent to me that Frost deserved a biography, and I decided that I would undertake the task.

Biographies come in many sorts. Some focus on the personal lives of public figures with well-known public lives. Others try to establish the place in history of someone not well known but important to the author. Others devote their pages to thoughtful analyses of the subject's work. Others are essentially prolonged eulogies. Similarly, the motivations of biographers are varied. Academic scholars often undertake such works, sometimes as outgrowths of graduate theses. A few fortunate authors are sufficiently well read to earn money from a published biography, especially when the subject is currently newsworthy.

What sort of biography is this? This book tells the little-known life story of a major academic medical figure. In doing so, it attempts to set his work in context and demonstrate its importance. It does not, however, provide a detailed analysis of Frost's published papers; interested readers should read these works themselves.

Why did I write this biography? Because Frost is a hero of mine, and his life should be better known to modern students of epidemiology and to the many who have benefitted from his work.

Acknowledgments

In preparing this work, I have had the generously given assistance of many persons. They have my gratitude, for I could not have completed this book without their help. More than that, they have my respect, for in helping me they revealed their own expertise in their various disciplines.

I must first acknowledge the Wade Hampton Frost Archives of the Claude Moore Health Sciences Library of the University of Virginia. This remarkable archive comprises Frost's personal papers and photographs donated by his daughter, Susan Frost Parrish; additional material donated by Jack M. Gwaltney Jr., Wade Hampton Frost Professor of Medicine Emeritus at the University of Virginia; and tape recordings of interviews of Frost's associates conducted by Barry M. Rutizer in 1975. Materials from this archive are reproduced with permission courtesy of the Historical Collection and Services of the Claude Moore Health Sciences Library. Joan Etchenkamp Klein, Assistant Director for Historical Collections and Services, welcomed me and facilitated my pursuit of Frost's life story in those archives. Joby Topper, Janet Pearson, and Hal Sharp of the Historical Collections staff gave me invaluable assistance. Dr. Gwaltney shared with me his insights into the life and important work of Frost.

Dr. Gwaltney and his gracious wife, Sarah, hosted me on several visits to the University of Virginia in Charlottesville, taking me and my wife in as guests in their home. Dr. Gwaltney also shared with me his extensive knowledge of the University of Virginia and of Frost's story. I obtained further information about Frost's Virginia years at Alderman Library of the University of Virginia, and I am grateful to the several librarians who assisted me there. Jeanne C. Pardee provided me with additional material from the Albert and Shirley Small Special Collections of that library. Alexander G. Gilliam Jr., Secretary of the Board of Visitors of the University of Virginia, kindly shared with me his knowledge of campus life at that university as it probably was during Frost's student days. Deborah Pugh of Special Collections at the McGraw-Page Library of Randolph-Macon College helped resolve conflicts in published accounts of Frost's attendance at that institution.

At the Johns Hopkins University Bloomberg School of Public Health, I received encouragement and support from George W. Comstock, Alumni Centennial Professor Emeritus of Epidemiology. Dr. Comstock is the leading epidemiologist of current times interested in tuberculosis and a long-time student of the life of Wade Hampton Frost. He provided me with numerous insights into Frost's life and kindly provided a foreword to this volume. He and Mrs. Comstock offered the hospitality of their home to me during my visit to them in Hagerstown, Maryland.

Jonathan Samet, Chairman of the Department of Epidemiology, kindly shared his views of the importance of Frost to the discipline of epidemiology with me. Charlotte Gerczak shared her extensive knowledge of the history of the Department of Epidemiology and of Frost's role in the early development of the department. She also graciously shared with me materials in the department and led me to other sources of information in the William Welch Medical Library. Additionally, Ms. Gerczak tirelessly answered my questions and researched information about the early days of the Department of Epidemiology in response to my many questions. At the Alan Mason Chesney Medical Archives of the Johns Hopkins Medical Institutions, Nancy McCall, archivist, and Gerard Shorb, research associate, welcomed me and provided me with access to material relevant to Frost.

John K. Gott of the Fauquier Heritage Society not only opened the archives of that society's library to me but spent hours with me discussing the history of Marshall, Virginia. He later reviewed my text concerning Marshall through several revisions, correcting many of my errors. Mary Ramey

Cunningham graciously talked with me at length about her memories of Marshall and allowed me to record our conversation.

Special mention should be made of Barry M. Rutizer, who tape-recorded the interviews mentioned above. At the time, he was a graduate student at the University of Virginia and was hired for this task. He has subsequently pursued a career as a journalist. Without his insightful interviews, the personal side of Frost would be unknown.

I have obtained much material from libraries in Cleveland, Ohio. The Allen Memorial and Health Sciences Libraries of Case Western Reserve University have extensive holdings in medical history, which I have consulted with great frequency, and I am indebted to Virginia Saha and James Edmondson of those libraries and the many members of their librarian staff who have assisted me. Similarly, the Kelvin Smith Library of Case Western Reserve University and its librarians have my gratitude. The Western Reserve Historical Society Library contains much useful genealogical information and, with the assistance of its kind and courteous staff, I was able to obtain additional information about the Frost, Walker, and Haxall families from its collections. Sharon Goolsby of the South Carolina School for the Deaf and Blind assisted me in my quest for information about the Walker family. The Center for Global Health and Diseases at Case Western Reserve University has provided space and office facilities for me, and April Rodon, the office assistant in that center, has provided important help in many ways from taking phone messages to unjamming the copier. A generous grant from the Division of Epidemiology and Virology of the Department of Medicine of the University of Virginia provided partial support for the preparation and publication of this book.

In documenting my sources, I have tried to be conscientious in all of my citations. I acknowledge, however, that I have confirmed details about the lives of many of Frost's associates in such standard reference works as *American Men and Women of Science* (in various editions), the *Directory of Medical Specialists*, directories of the American Medical Association and

American College of Physicians, the *Directory of Deceased American Physicians of the American Medical Association*, the *Official List of Commissioned and Other Officers of the United States Public Health Service*, and similar works. I have not always specifically cited these reference works.

Perhaps my greatest debt of all is to my wife of more than fifty years, Janet S. Daniel. She has comforted and encouraged me throughout my career in academic medicine and at every step along the way of this sometimes joyful, sometimes tedious project. She spent countless hours standing at a copying machine duplicating pages I selected. She has read and reread every word and page of this book through numerous versions and revisions, finding errors and making helpful suggestions that have clarified and improved my presentation. Without her, my career would have been vastly different, and this book would not have been written.

1

By What Name?

By him we shall be judged.
— *Wade Hampton Frost*[1]

"By what name shall this child be called?"

The sun streamed in through the window of Trinity Church in Marshall, Virginia. It was a warm Sunday morning in 1880. Dr. Henry Frost was lost in reverie, his mind wandering in the past and paying scant attention to the words of the minister who was about to baptize his seventh child. Perhaps he was tired from an all-night vigil with a dying patient. Again, the minister's voice intoned, "By what name . . ."

"Wade Hampton," said the father, starting from his inattention and speaking the name of the confederate general under whom he had served and to whom his mind had strayed during the service. Thus did Wade Hampton Frost acquire his name. Or so it was repeatedly told in the Frost family.[2]

Or perhaps, one might suppose, Henry Frost really did intend to name his son for the Civil War confederate hero. What might that have meant to the father? And what might it later have meant to the son? Wade Hampton was the most famous South Carolinian of the time.[3] A big, handsome, imposing man, an enormously wealthy cotton plantation owner, an expert horseman facile with weapons of the hunt, Wade Hampton was not a secessionist, but when the Civil War erupted he accepted a commission and quickly raised a legion of his fellow citizens of South Carolina. He trained these men and led them north to the front, where they distinguished themselves, as did he, often outperforming the gray-clad troops led by other confederate officers who had learned their military command skills at West Point. Ultimately, Wade Hampton was promoted to lieutenant general and served in command of all of the confederate cavalry forces. He led his troops, Henry Frost among them, from the front of the battle, and was loved by them. At the Battle of Gettysburg he was severely wounded and evacuated first to Charlottesville, Virginia, and later to his home in South Carolina. Although he is sometimes portrayed as sterner than other confederate officers, a letter to his wife commenting on a deep head wound reveals a whimsical sense of humor.

> The penitentiary style in which my hair is cut, half the head being shaven, is striking if not beautiful. It suits all kind of weather, as one side of my head is sure to be just right, either for cool, or for hot weather. But the flies play the mischief, as they wander over the bald side.[4]

Wade Hampton recovered from his wounds and returned to the front lines in Virginia. As Sherman marched his rampaging forces through the South, Hampton returned to the area to engage them. After the war Hampton was penniless, holding land that had been sacked and could not be worked profitably. Despite this, he emerged as the leader of South Carolina and much of the South during the reconstruction era. After a fractious election, he became governor of South Carolina in November 1876. The following February he resigned the governorship to represent South Carolina as a United States senator, and he was serving in that position at the time Henry Frost named his son for him. He retired from the Senate at the end of 1892 and died of heart failure on April 1, 1902.

Henry Frost, the father of the new infant, was born in Charleston, South Carolina, on November 2, 1839. He graduated from South Carolina College in 1859 and then attended the South Carolina Medical College, graduating in 1861. With the outbreak of war, he enlisted in Wade Hampton's corps, initially in the artillery, but soon as an assistant surgeon. In 1864 he married Sabra Jane Walker of Spartanburg, South Carolina. At the war's end he returned to his ravaged home state and tried for two years to establish a practice of medicine. Unsuccessful, he decided to move to northern Virginia, an area in which he must have seen military action under Hampton. He entrusted his savings to a friend who offered to buy land for him, but what the friend bought turned out to be a non-arable "rock pile," poor land—mostly gravel with little top soil.[5]

Unaware of what lay ahead but determined to escape the apparently futureless Charleston and Spartanburg, Frost took his wife and first child north to Fauquier County, Virginia, initially settling on the land his friend had purchased for him near Delaplane. He was unable to establish a profitable medical practice there, and so he farmed as best he could and as the land permitted. He struggled to put food on the table. In 1872 he moved to nearby Marshall, Virginia, less than twenty miles from Manassas where Hampton's men first saw military action. There he met with success, raised his family, and practiced medicine until his death in 1917.[6]

Wade Hampton Frost was interested in his South Carolina roots. Did his famous namesake create a mandate for him? A mandate of service? A mandate of courtly or patrician behavior? A mandate to adhere to principles without compromise? A mandate to overcome adversity? Did his father, with whom he had a close relationship in boyhood and with whom he corresponded as he grew into adulthood, think of the name as a potential molder of the boy? Did Frost himself feel he should fit the Hampton mold? We shall see that much in Wade Hampton Frost's life might have drawn guidance from the heroic image of General Wade Hampton.

Yet, we must not forget that Wade Hampton Frost, who was always called Wade by his family and in Marshall, was known to his wife and many close friends by the puckish nickname of "Jack."

2

Origins

Papa is kept so busy that he can seldom write
to me.

—*Wade Hampton Frost*[1]

Wade Hampton Frost was greatly interested in his ancestry, and his antecedents certainly had more than casual meaning for him. He corresponded with relatives in South Carolina, in England, and elsewhere to piece together his family tree. In fact, the Frost family was a prominent one in South Carolina, and Frost was able to collect published accounts of his forebears as well as pedigrees. Figure 2.1 illustrates this interest. It is a family tree in Frost's handwriting tracing his ancestry back through his paternal grandmother, Mary Deas Lesesne (1807–1866), who married Henry Rutledge Frost, a prominent physician in Charleston, South Carolina. Three prior generations carried this lineage back to John Deas (1735–1790). Frost's wife, Susan, shared his interest, and she penciled notes on some of the documents he assembled.

Through correspondence with Horace C. Frost, a distant relative living in England, Frost was able to obtain a pedigree of the Frost family beginning with John Frost, who lived in the late fourteenth and early fifteenth centuries in Pulham, Norfolk County, England, and extending through nine generations to Thomas Frost, who emigrated from England to South Carolina in 1785.[2] There were five early colonists named Frost who left England for the new world, most of them not closely related. Thomas Frost was the last to arrive.[3] His lineage to Wade Hampton Frost is well documented, and it is of interest to us—as it certainly was to Frost—to consider who these early American Frost forebears were and what sort of men and women they were. They were well educated. They were productive

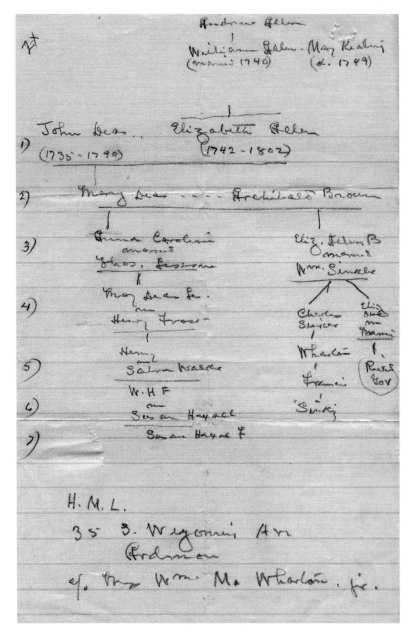

Figure 2.1. Family tree of Frost genealogy drawn by Wade Hampton Frost. Claude Moore Health Sciences Library, University of Virginia Health Sciences Center, Charlottesville, VA: Wade Hampton Frost Archives, Box 5, Folder 16. Reproduced with permission, courtesy of the Historical Collection and Services of the Claude Moore Health Sciences Library.

citizens. They were leading members of their churches. They were steeped in a growing family tradition of service. Wade Hampton Frost's great grandfather was a clergyman. His grandfather was a leading physician of his times and a professor of medicine specializing in pharmacology. His father was a much loved physician devoted to the care of his patients and also a founder of his local county medical society.

The first member of the Frost line in America was Thomas Frost, born in 1758 in England. He studied for the ministry at Caius College, Cambridge. Although he seemed not to take his studies seriously at the time, he nevertheless received his degree with honors. In 1870 he won a prize at Caius College as "the student standing highest among his fellows . . . in the philosophical schools." He was a spendthrift, living beyond his means and incurring debts for his parents. As a university student, he was known as "Jolly" Frost. His surgeon father urged him to emigrate to America and may have helped pay for his passage, hoping thus to free himself of the problems created by his son's profligacy. Little effort was made by Frost or his parents to communicate or maintain contact after his emigration, and a coolness between the English and American branches of the Frost family persisted through several generations.[4]

Thomas Frost arrived in Charleston, South Carolina, in 1785. On November 15, 1787 he married Elizabeth Downes, a woman of some wealth who was descended from Francis LeJau, a prominent French Huguenot clergyman.[5] Frost attempted to establish a brickyard; this venture failed, and it cost much of his wife's property to settle the debts incurred. Subsequently he found a position as rector at St. Philip's Episcopal Church; the date of this appointment is not clear, but he is first recorded as having officiated at a wedding in the church on June 6, 1798.[6] He did well in this position and was much beloved in the community. After his death, he was eulogized as

> a worthy clergyman. [As] a husband and father, . . . he will be ranked among those who have excelled. . . . In the dignified station of a

Minister of the Gospel of Christ, his conduct was exemplary—he
loved his flock. . . . As a preacher he was eminently great; his doctrine
was sound and catholic, his style pure.[7]

But however he may have excelled as a clergyman, Thomas
Frost was not a paragon of a breadwinner and family supporter.
His profligacy remained unchecked, and his wife struggled to
put bread on the table and to educate their children.

Thomas Frost died at the age of forty-six in 1804. His early
death left his wife with four children, the youngest of whom
was only two. She apparently did not remarry, but she
managed to hold the family together and launch her children
onto successful lives. Her grandson is reported to have said, "if
any merit were ever discovered in our family, it was due to
[Elizabeth Downes Frost]"[8] In fact, the children of Elizabeth
and Thomas Frost did well. Their first son, Thomas, followed
his father into the ministry. It was said in Charleston that the
parishioners of St. Philip's were "Frost-bitten."[9] Their second
son, Henry Rutledge Frost studied medicine at the University
of Pennsylvania. A daughter, Ellen Legare Frost, married
Thomas Parker and raised a family of seven children, one of
whom, Francis LeJau Parker, studied medicine at the Medical
College of South Carolina and then apprenticed himself to
his uncle, Henry Rutledge Frost.[10] Edward Frost, the youngest
of the boys, attended Yale University, became a lawyer and
judge, and served in the state legislature.[11] One of his sons,
Francis LeJau Frost, studied medicine and practiced in
Charleston.[12]

Henry Rutledge Frost, the second son of Thomas Frost and
Elizabeth Downes Frost and grandfather of Wade Hampton
Frost, was born in Charleston on October 6, 1795. He was a nine
year-old youngster when his father died. After a period of
schooling at Dr. Waddell's Academy in Wilmington, North
Carolina, he returned to Charleston to begin medical studies as
an apprentice to Dr. Philip G. Prioleau, embarking thus on the
usual course of education of that time for individuals wishing
to become physicians.[13] He then attended the medical school
of the University of Pennsylvania in Philadelphia, receiving his
doctor of Medicine degree in 1816. He remained in Philadelphia

for two more years as a resident physician at the Philadelphia Alms House. Frost returned to Charleston in 1818 and began a general practice at the Shirras Dispensary.[14]

Henry Rutledge Frost became interested in what was then termed "materia medica," the discipline we now know as pharmacology. He wrote papers on this subject and began offering lectures in this field. He became particularly interested in the pharmacologic effects of tobacco, feeling it to be detrimental to health, with its action mediated largely by absorption through the mucosa of the nose. Beginning in December 1821, Frost joined with several of his Charleston medical colleagues in promoting the establishment of a medical school in that city. As a result of these efforts, the Medical College of South Carolina was founded in November 1824 with seven faculty members. Henry Rutledge Frost assumed the chair of materia medica and later served two terms as the dean of the school. Students were required to have served three years of medical apprenticeship and then to attend the lectures of the medical school for two years. In fact, in the spring of 1823 Frost and the others had begun giving lectures, which then were accepted as part of the course of study for the first students. The first commencement was held on April 4, 1825, with five graduates receiving their degrees.[15]

As a professor, Frost was scholarly but not inspiring. He was a poor lecturer, handicapped by "a modesty that amounted to diffidence."[16] He published a pharmacology text described by one historian as "rather dull, but what materia medica is not."[17] As a physician, Frost was caring, devoted to his patients, and much beloved. "His leading traits were mildness, kind-heartedness, benevolence, and an indefatigable zeal in the discharge of his duties. . . ."[18] As a man, Frost was devoted to public service and a committed member of his church, where he served as a vestryman for many years.[19]

Henry Rutledge Frost married Mary Deas Lesesne, seven years his junior, probably in the mid 1830s. They had six children. Their second born was Henry Frost, father of Wade Hampton Frost. Late in his life, Henry Rutledge Frost served briefly in the Confederate army as an assistant surgeon. He died on April 7, 1866; the cause of death was said to have been diarrhea.[20] His wife died in the same year.

Henry Frost, Wade Hampton Frost's father, was born on November 2, 1839. He attended the South Carolina College, graduating in 1859, and in 1861 he received a Doctor of Medicine degree from South Carolina Medical College in Charleston. With the outbreak of the Civil War, he joined the corps of Wade Hampton and served as an assistant surgeon, as noted in chapter 1. After the war, he tried to practice medicine in Charleston and in Spartanburg, South Carolina, but the reconstruction period was one of great economic depression, and Frost found it difficult to become established. He married Sabra Jane Walker of Spartanburg, South Carolina, in 1864. The couple's first child, Mary Deas Frost, was born on August 9, 1866.

Sabra Jane Walker was the daughter of Reverend Newton Pinckney Walker. Reverend Walker was born in Spartanburg, South Carolina, on November 29, 1816. Little is known of his antecedents or his early life. He grew up at Cedar Spring, four miles south of Spartanburg and became a teacher and Baptist minister. Walker married Martha Louise Hughston, whose family had a farm at Cedar Spring. They had three sons and four daughters, one of whom was Sabra Jane. Three of Martha Louise (Hughston) Walker's brothers were deaf, and the couple decided something should be done for them. In 1848, after Walker had visited a school for the deaf at Cave Spring in Georgia to observe its techniques, he and his wife opened a school for five deaf individuals in their home. Three of the students were Martha's siblings; two were other Spartanburg residents. Walker then purchased the delapidated Cedar Spring Hotel and its one hundred and fifty acres of land.

After making building repairs, the couple opened what soon became known locally as the Walker's Mute School or the Cedar Spring Asylum in January 1849. Garnering support and funds from the State of South Carolina, it became the South Carolina School for the Deaf and Blind in 1859. Although closed for some time during the post Civil War Reconstruction, it reopened and continues to this day as a premier education facility for individuals thus handicapped. Walker died in 1861.

Martha stepped forward and continued the school. Her son, Newton Farmer Walker, who was then eighteen, returned from the Confederate army to assist her; he later became the school's superintendent, serving in this capacity until he died at age eighty-two. Henry Frost volunteered his medical services at his in-laws' school.[21]

Sabra Jane Walker was born on December 22, 1839. Nothing is known of her education, but it can be presumed she was well schooled, for she knew and later taught both Latin and Greek. Her younger brother, Newton Farmer Walker, attended the Cedar Springs Academy and St. John's Classical and Military School in Spartanburg; he had planned to attend college, but enlisted in the Confederate army instead. One can presume that Sabra was similarly educated, perhaps at the Girls Academy of Cedar Spring.

South Carolina was devastated and racked by the corruption and violence that marked the early reconstruction years. Income from the practice of medicine there at that time was insufficient to meet the Frosts' needs. Payment of doctors during those times was difficult for all South Carolinians. In Spartanburg Henry Frost made *pro bono* professional visits to his father-in-law's school, donating his services without compensation. Especially after the death of both of his parents in 1866, there seemed little point in remaining in his home state. Sabra Walker Frost's father had died in 1861; her ties to Spartanburg were weak, and she would gladly follow her husband. Now married and a father, Frost recalled northern Virginia, where he had served with Hampton's forces during the war, and so in 1866, as we saw in chapter 1, he and his young family moved to Fauquier County, Virginia, initially settling near Delaplane. Ties with South Carolina remained, however. Sabra Walker Frost returned to Spartanburg for the birth of Henry Pinckney Frost, their second child, on October 10, 1868.[22] Like his father and younger brother, he studied medicine, becoming a neurologist and practicing at mental hospitals in Buffalo, New York, and Boston, Massachusetts.

Northern Virginia, including Fauquier County, had been the scene of many Civil War battles. However, it had not suffered the widespread ravaging that Sherman's troops had inflicted on the cities of South Carolina and Georgia. The transition from slavery-based to share cropper or employee-based agriculture was made with relative peace, although it resulted in contraction of most agricultural holdings. There was widespread political apathy, with only a small minority of individuals exercising their franchise.[23] In this environment small farms developed from former large holdings, and the small farming communities of Fauquier County were at least stable, although titles to land were somewhat vague. Most of the land was not fertile, more suitable for grazing than growing crops. Farming was difficult and usually not prosperous. The farm that Henry Frost bought near Cool Springs Church in Delaplane barely supported his family as he struggled to establish himself as a physician in the impoverished community. The Frosts were, in the words of one older Fauquier County resident who remembers the Frost family, "dirt poor."[24] Two more children, both daughters, were born to Henry and Sabra Frost during the Delaplane years. Martha Louisa Frost was born on December 28, 1870 and Anna Lesesne Frost on March 31, 1872.

In 1872, Frost moved to Marshall where he prospered and was loved in the community. There Henry and Sabra Frost raised their family, including Wade Hampton Frost, their seventh child and third son.

3

Marshall

We sat around and talked a while about "old
times."

—*Wade Hampton Frost*[1]

At the end of the nineteenth century, Marshall, Virginia, was a
one-street town, as it largely remains today. For about one mile
on the road between Delaplane to the west and The Plains to
the east, one-half acre lots faced each other across Main Street.
Main Street was narrow and unpaved, but gracious and lined
with mature shade trees. Most of the houses and buildings had
porches, many ornately carved with latticed railings in the
then-fashionable Victorian style. The trees and porches have
long since been lost, fallen to the widening and paving of what
is now Virginia Route 55.

At the east edge of the town, Rectortown Road ran to the
north, with only two houses on it. To the south at the same
point the Warrenton Road had two buildings facing each other,
Trinity Episcopal Church on the east side of the road and the
Salem Academy on the west. This latter building housed a
school; it was originally built in 1771 as a Baptist meeting
house, and the Baptist graveyard served as the playground for
the school. East of Marshall was a community known as
Rosstown settled by former slaves freed after the Civil War.[2]

Marshall was chartered by the General Assembly of Virginia
on December 14, 1796, as Salem. To avoid confusion with
another, larger Salem in Roanoke County, the postoffice referred
to the town as Salem-Fauquier, a cumbersome designation
never used by the villagers. At the insistence of the postal
authorities, the townspeople met in December 1881 to choose a
new name for the town. As he was about to leave for the meeting, Philip Klipstein, one of the town's leading businessmen and

a descendant of a Hessian soldier who had remained in Virginia after his Revolutionary War capture, asked his wife if she had suggestions for a name. She suggested the name of Marshall, honoring Supreme Court Chief Justice John Marshall, whose home was three miles west of the town. Klipstein offered the suggestion at the town meeting, where it was accepted, and the demands of the postal authorities were met. On March 9, 1882, the name change became official. Fauquier County, in which Marshall sits, had been named for Francis Fauquier, Lieutenant Governor of Virginia, in 1759.

To the west and southwest of Marshall was an area known as the Free State. Historically the "Northern Neck" of Virginia comprised all the territory between the Potomac and Rappahannock Rivers from their headsprings to Chesapeake Bay. This vast area had been granted by exiled King Charles II of England to seven of his loyal followers. Through purchase and inheritance this proprietary came into the possession of the Fairfax family of Leeds Castle under the English system known as freehold tenure. For a quit-rent of one shilling for each fifty acres, the Fairfaxes held hereditary effective title to the entire area with rights to sublease land as they desired, although nominal ownership of the land remained with the English sovereign. The Reverend Denny Martin Fairfax, heir of his uncle, Thomas, Sixth Lord of Fairfax, came to Virginia in 1797 in an attempt to protect his inheritance. With the legal assistance of John Marshall, later Chief Justice of the United States, he secured sole title to 220,000 acres from his many claimant relatives. Ultimately, John Marshall, his brother, and brother-in-law purchased this vast holding, known as the Manor of Leeds, from Fairfax for the sum of twenty thousand pounds.[3]

Following American independence, land titles in the Free State were poorly understood and frequently contested by local residents. Many small landholders whose families had farmed their acreage for generations refused to pay rent to the Marshall family landlords; they felt they owned the land. On the other hand, when tax collectors appeared, they often refused to pay taxes and claimed to be merely Marshall tenants.[4]

Although not the county seat, Marshall, the oldest town in Fauquier County, was known as "the capital of the Free State" in the late nineteenth century. It was the commercial center. John Martin Ramey and Major Thomas Redmond Foster operated general stores; William D. Maddux a hotel with an adjoining barroom attended by his son-in-law, Thomas S. Johnson; Mrs. Moses M. Gibson a millinery where fine ladies' fashions were offered. The post office was located in Ramey's store. Mail was sorted alphabetically and left for the intended recipients in sections of a wooden frame hanging on the wall. Figure 3.1 shows Main Street as it looked in 1915; the photograph was taken looking west from the location of Ramey's store. Philip Augustus Klipstein, whose wife suggested the town's name, operated a chemical factory at the west end of Marshall, the only industry in the community. There a number of household products were made, including Carbona (carbon tetrachloride), a cleaning solvent widely distributed and popular

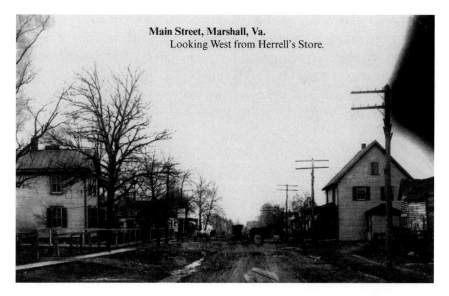

Main Street, Marshall, Va.
Looking West from Herrell's Store.

Figure 3.1. Main Street of Marshall, Virginia, in 1915. This photograph was taken from the location of Ramey's Store (later renamed Herrell's Store) and looks to the west. Courtesy of John K. Gott, Fauquier Heritage Society, Marshall, Virginia. Reproduced with permission.

because it was not flammable. Carbon tetrachloride fumes are toxic, however, and it is no longer in use. Major Foster, one of the town's wealthiest citizens, purchased much of the land both east and west of Marshall, including substantial amounts owned by Klipstein, who was deeply in debt following the Civil War. The railroad station was situated at one end of Foster's store east of the town. There were Baptist, Episcopal, Presbyterian, and Methodist churches in Marshall.

Rich blue grass country surrounded Marshall, and today rich estates and prosperous horse barns and pastures still characterize the rolling green hills and low mountains of the area. Cattle-raising was the principal commerce of this lush region, and Marshall families such as the Rameys and Fosters had farms with large herds of cattle. Occasionally these animals were driven through town to the cattle pens adjacent to the railroad station. Smaller farms in the Free State raised turkeys and each fall the town witnessed drives of several hundred turkeys raised on these farms. Chestnuts gathered in the forests were another product of the Free State, and six-horse-wagon loads of these nuts traversed Main Street in the fall. Both the birds and the nuts were due for shipment by rail to eastern American cities to become part of winter holiday celebrations.

There was a frontier town atmosphere about Marshall. Free Staters were a rough bunch. When Free Staters were in town, women and children remained inside with doors closed and windows shuttered. Street fights were commonplace, many of them centered at or near Rector's livery stable, the loft of which served as the local gambling house and brothel for the Free Staters.

The "saloon era" in Marshall ended abruptly in 1887. Reverend James Grammar of Trinity Episcopal Church, who disapproved not only of saloons but of dancing, card playing, and the circus, led a temperance campaign. With his encouragement, church women held prayer and hymn-singing vigils in the streets outside of drinking establishments. The ladies of Marshall's Baptist, Methodist, and Presbyterian churches were joined by Episcopalian women. On June 2, 1887, Judge

Edward Spilman from his court in Warrenton refused to renew the license of Presley N. Lawrence, who operated the last remaining barroom in Marshall.[5]

In 1872 Clement Coote Spieden was the only doctor in Marshall. He was highly respected for his skill in extracting bullets and suturing knife wounds. He left Marshall in that year, however, to join his brother-in-law, who was building a railroad in Costa Rica. Major Foster sought out Henry Frost and induced him to leave the infertile and nonproductive farm he owned near Delaplane and move to Marshall to assume the departing man's general practice and become the new physician in the town. Foster had planned to build a house on Main Street just east of the Warrenton Road in a tree-shaded area known as "The Grove" for his daughter. However, she and her husband moved to Richmond about that time. Foster then built the house for Frost and sold it to him. Frost also acquired a small adjacent building as an office. Thus, in 1872, Henry Frost became Marshall's only doctor. He would serve the community throughout the remainder of his life. He rapidly established a successful, if not highly remunerative practice; doctors in rural Virginia at that time were more often paid with hams, chickens, or produce than with cash. For years thereafter, however, Henry Frost and his family made occasional pilgrimages to Delaplane where their life as Virginians began.

Henry Frost was beloved. No one else in Marshall at that time was held in such esteem and was so revered. A friend eulogized him at the time of his death, praising his skill—"He has never been known to make a wrong diagnosis"—and his compassion—"I have known of his pushing the hard-earned fee back into a poor woman's hand, saying, 'Keep it; you need it more than I do.'"[6] A long term resident of Marshall refused to seek medical attention late in her life. She kept a picture of Dr. Henry Frost hanging in her bedroom. "That dear old face is all the medicine I need to get me through the day," she said. Frost sometimes spent the night at the bedside of gravely ill or dying patients. His horse was well trained, so that late on a winter night he could climb into his buggy, wrap himself in oilcloth with a brick warmed on his patient's stove at his feet, and drop the reins; the horse knew the way home.[7]

Henry and Sabra Frost were respected and admired in Marshall. They were cultured and educated. If Marshall could be said to have had an aristocracy, the Frosts were part of it. Years later, the nameless street crossing Marshall's main thoroughfare was named Frost Street to honor the doctor who had served the community so well and for so long. Many children were given names that included Frost as homage to the doctor who had brought them into the world. Figure 3.2 is a photograph of Henry Frost.

Frost's medical practice included the full range of actions expected of doctors at that time. Marshall had a dentist, so he did not have to deal with toothaches, nor did he prescribe glasses. But he performed what surgery could be done on a kitchen table, delivered babies, managed broken bones and other trauma, and cared for the illnesses that occurred among the townspeople of Marshall. He charged his patients $2.50 for a house call.[8] Pneumonia, tuberculosis, and diarrheal diseases were the three leading causes of death in the United States in 1910, and it is certain they were prominent among the ills of Frost's patients. There were also more than 175,000 cases of diphtheria in America in that year, and nearly 150,000 cases of whooping cough; Frost and his patients knew those diseases as well.[9]

Henry Frost was respected not only by his patients but also by his Virginia professional peers and colleagues. In 1889 he was president of the Northeast Virginia Medical Society, originally founded ten years earlier as the Fauquier County Medical Society.[10]

There was no pharmacy in the village, so Frost obtained drugs from Warrenton to supply to his patients. His bag and his office shelf would have included ether, morphine, digitalis, diphtheria antitoxin, smallpox vaccine, iron, quinine, iodine, alcohol, and mercury.[11] He had his office in a two-story building—one room on the first floor, one room above—next door to his house. The office occupied the first floor room; it was comfortably furnished and had a fireplace providing warmth.

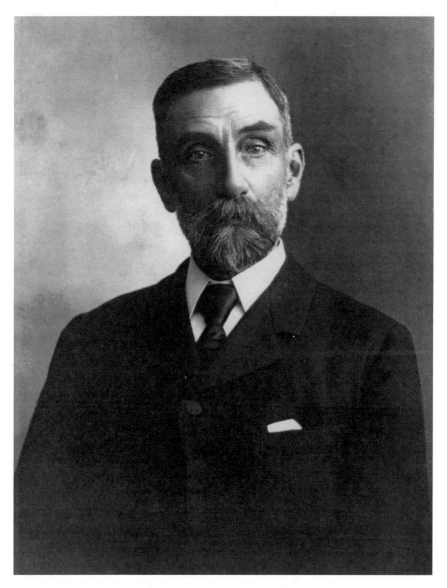

Figure 3.2. Henry Frost. The date of this photograph is unknown. Courtesy of John K. Gott, Fauquier Heritage Society, Marshall, Virginia. Reproduced with permission.

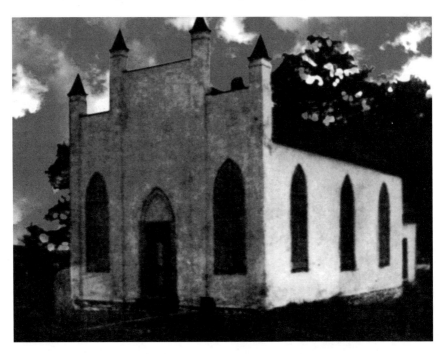

Figure 3.3. Trinity Episcopal Church as it appeared during the years it was attended by the Frost family. The church was originally erected about 1848. Later a steeple was erected by John T. Ramey, Wade Hampton Frost's boyhood friend, in memory of Ramey's deceased wife, Jane Mason Ramey, substantially changing its appearance. Courtesy of John K. Gott, Fauquier Heritage Society, Marshall, Virginia. Reproduced with permission.

Henry Frost was a devout member of Trinity Episcopal Church on Warrenton Road just around the corner from his house. He taught Sunday School and served as a vestryman for thirty years. Much of the Frost family and social life centered around the church. Figure 3.3, taken from a contemporaneous post card, shows Trinity Church at it appeared at that time.

The Frost house still stands today on East Main Street, largely unchanged from the time when the Frost family occupied it. Figure 3.4 shows it in 2001. By today's standards it is small for a family with eight children. On the first floor a center hall is flanked by a living room and parlor. Behind the living room is a dining room, and behind it a kitchen in an el. On the second floor there are three bedrooms. Over the kitchen is a small

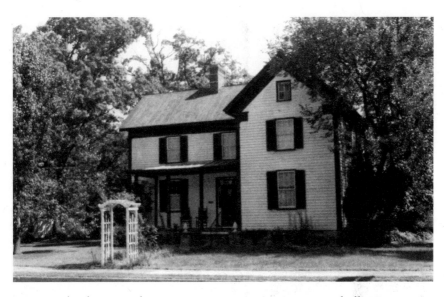

Figure 3.4. The Frost house on East Main Street in Marshall, Virginia, in 2001. It is essentially unchanged in appearance from the time when it was occupied by the Frost family. Photograph by the author.

room probably intended for a servant. Although the Frosts hired a cook, she lived in Rosstown, and the room over the kitchen provided sleeping quarters for a child. The Frost sons slept next door in the room above Frost's medical office.

The Frost family grew. Mary Deas had been born in Spartanburg, South Carolina; Henry Pinckney, Martha Louise, and Anna Lesesne while the Frosts lived in Delaplane. Four more children followed: Thomas Lownes Frost was born on October 28, 1874; Harriet Frost on June 18, 1877; Wade Hampton Frost on March 3, 1880; and James Henderson Frost on July 24, 1882.[12] The oldest daughter, Mary Deas Frost, died of tuberculosis on March 4, 1904. Henry Pinckney Frost, who had tuberculosis as a youngster but recovered from the illness, studied medicine at the University of Maryland and became a neuropsychiatrist. He died on May 23, 1917 in Boston, Massachusetts, where he was the director of the Mattapan State Hospital. His death was recorded as due to pneumonia, but family members thought he had a brain tumor or meningitis. One must wonder if he might have developed fatal tuberculous meningitis as a consequence of relapse of his earlier disease. None of the Frost daughters married. Martha Louise Frost, known as Mattie, remained in Marshall with the Frost family, providing care for her parents in their later years. After their deaths, she moved to Philadelphia and lived with her sisters. She died on August 16, 1956. Anna Lesesne Frost, usually called Ann, and Harriet Frost, known as Hallie, both became nurses in Philadelphia. They died on September 9, 1953, and March 9, 1962, respectively. Thomas Lownes Frost was a successful accountant initially in New York City, later in Marshall. His life was cut short by tuberculosis, to which he succumbed on March 16, 1923, leaving a wife and three children, one of whom, also named Tom, went on to serve in the Virginia state legislature. The youngest son of Henry and Sabra Frost, James Henderson, remained in Marshall throughout his life until his death on December 22, 1935. He worked as a clerk in E. S. Renald's store, located in the old Foster store building at the railroad. All of the Frost children were intelligent—James, the youngest, less so. Several pursued higher education and achieved professional success, two sons as physicians, two daughters as nurses. Figure 3.5 shows the Frost family on the front steps of their home in Marshall in 1907.

In the late nineteenth-century years of Wade Hampton Frost's boyhood, the quality of schools in Fauquier County did not meet the standards of the Frost family. Salem Academy had been founded in 1809 as a private school in the building originally built as a Baptist meeting house. It became a public school in 1871. However, the Frosts and many of their neighbors were dissatisfied with it. But if public schools were inadequate, that did not mean that children were not to be properly educated. The responsibility for teaching them not just manners but reading and mathematics and literature—all of the many things a young Virginian should know—then fell on mothers. Sabra Walker Frost took on this job with a cheerful heart, not only for her own children but also for a class of as many as twenty other children of Marshall, The Plains, and Middleburg. Assisted by her daughter, Anna, she conducted

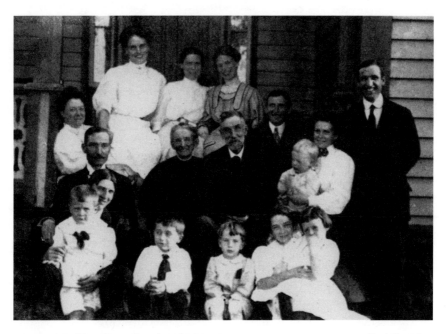

Figure 3.5. The Frost family in 1907. Front row: James H. Frost, holding his nephew, Tom Frost (son of Thomas L. and Elizabeth Frost); Henry, Pinckney, and Virginia Frost (children of Henry Pinckney and Margaret Frost); Elizabeth Frost (daughter of Thomas L. and Elizabeth Frost). Second row: Henry Pinckney Frost; Sabra Jane Walker Frost; Henry Frost; Thomas L. Frost; Elizabeth Frost (wife of Thomas L. Frost) holding her son Robert; Wade Hampton Frost. Back row: Margaret Frost (wife of Henry Pinckney Frost); Harriet Frost; Anna Lesesne Frost; Martha Louise Frost. Photograph courtesy of John K. Gott, Fauquier Heritage Society, Marshall, Virginia. Reproduced with permission.

school in her home, and she was a talented teacher. She used the McGuffey readers, but her curriculum also included music, mathematics, classical civilizations, and Latin and French. Sabra Walker Frost was much loved and respected in the community and by her students for this effort.[13] After her death, one of her former pupils, Thomas R. Foster, wrote:

My first day at school made an impression on me that is still remembered. I had come in and gone through some examination as to what I knew, and been assigned a lesson to study. Having no desk, I was allowed to stand at the open window while studying, but I became much more interested in the efforts of Jim Frost to get a wheelbarrow load of wood over a little rise than in my book, and, finally, forgetting where I was, I began shouting encouragement at the top of my lungs. I don't remember what Mrs. Frost said, but though she was very gentle, her words, and the laughter of the other children, imprinted the incident in my memory.

   She taught me more than anyone else was able to get into my head, and we all loved her as a teacher is seldom loved by her pupils.[14]

Sabra Walker Frost was talented, intelligent, and well educated. In the photograph reproduced in figure 3.6 she chose to pose holding a book or magazine. She also had a gentle sense of humor. Fearing that her cook was stealing flour from the flour barrel in the kitchen, she took to writing phrases in Latin in the surface of the flour. Her script would be disturbed when flour was removed. The cook could not read English, much less Latin, but it pleased Sabra Frost to use the esoteric language.

There came a time when the ravages of age and illness encroached upon the active lives of Henry and Sabra Frost. Their unmarried daughter Mattie (Martha Louise Frost) lived with them and provided care for them. Henry Frost suffered from peripheral vascular disease—arteriosclerosis affecting the arteries carrying blood to his legs—and developed gangrene of his toes and feet. He underwent an amputation, but continued to teach Sunday school and see some of his long-time patients. He was joined in Marshall by Dr. Thomas Flatford Gill, who lessened his clinical load. Gill later became a successful physician in Richmond, Virginia. In 1914, then seventy-five years old, Henry Frost wrote to his son, Wade Hampton, who was stationed in Cincinnati. At the time he was probably convalescing from the amputation, getting about on crutches:

   I have almost nothing to do, and when I propose to do anything, they [his wife and daughter] persuade me not to do it. . . . I have really improved very much lately, but still tire easily if I try to walk much, [but] I don't walk much. I have very little to do: a few office patients and an occasional call to which I have to sneak off.[15]

Letters written in November and early December of 1915 speak of the failing health of Sabra Walker Frost. She suffered

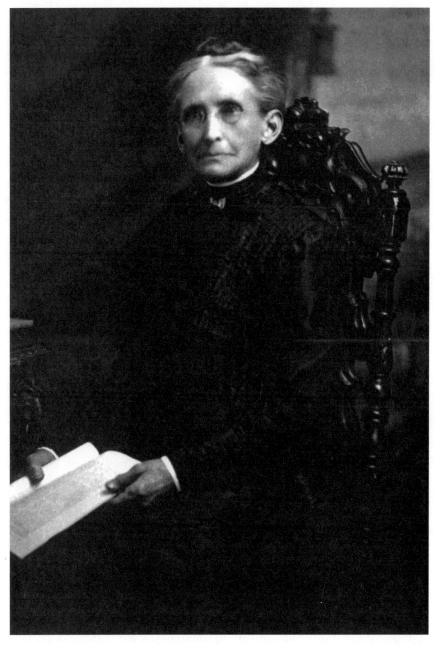

Figure 3.6. Sabra Jane Walker Frost. The date of this photograph is unknown. Courtesy of John K. Gott, Fauquier Heritage Society, Marshall, Virginia. Reproduced with permission, courtesy of the Historical Collection and Services of the Claude Moore Health Sciences Library.

from major rectal bleeding. Henry Frost treated her for bleeding hemorrhoids and was concerned that she might have a colonic cancer. To the modern medical reader his account also suggests bleeding from diverticulosis. In April of 1916 Sabra Frost was apparently improved, but Henry Frost was developing gangrene in the toes of his remaining leg. The fall of that year and the spring of 1917 found him in Philadelphia at the Orthopedic Hospital, where his daughter, Anna Lesesne Frost, was on the nursing staff, with the threat of a second amputation looming.[16]

Henry Frost died in Philadelphia on March 23, 1917. Sabra Walker Frost died on April 27, 1917. Henry and Sabra Frost had been born only one month apart in 1839. They followed one another in death by a similar short interval at age 78. They lie together in the Marshall cemetery, surrounded by all of their children except Wade Hampton Frost.

Wade Hampton Frost was the seventh child of that remarkable couple. The only published description of him as a boy is that of Kenneth F. Maxcy, his colleague at Johns Hopkins, who assembled a posthumous collection of Frost's major scientific publications. He included a biographical introduction to which Frost's sister Harriet was a major (although unacknowledged) contributor.[17] Maxcy described the young Frost as:

> Naturally thoughtful and studious . . . rather dreamy, but stoutly aggressive when his indignation was aroused, . . . a voracious reader of the few but choice books that were available in his home. His favorite was John Bunyan's *Pilgrim's Progress*.[18]

Frost's boyhood friend, John T. Ramey, remembered him warmly. "As a young man the thoughtful and idealistic side of his nature was balanced by a remarkably gay and happy one which endeared him to young and old."[19] Mary Cunningham, a long-time Marshall resident and Ramey's daughter, who knew all of the Frost family, had a distinctly different picture of the young boy.

> As a boy growing up, he was full of fun, full of mischief. . . . He had a marvelous sense of humor and was very clever.[20]

Cunningham thinks of Frost not only as a fun-loving youngster but also as part of a family whose life centered around intellectual activities. Not oriented to social status, the Frost family members placed high value on cerebral activities.

> They were all clever. The whole family, except the youngest one, was clever. They were clever at writing. They were clever in their thinking. They were very education-minded, the whole family. They were literary people. They were students.[21]

The fun-loving side of the young Frost is revealed in anecdotes well known in Marshall. There being no janitors in churches in Marshall at the time, the young members of the Frost family helped to clean the four churches in the village on Saturdays. While the girls dusted the pulpit and other items in the sanctuary, the boys cleaned the pews by sliding from one end to the other, pants serving as cleaning cloths. Their mother is said to have been tolerant of this approach to cleanliness.[22]

The Reverend James Grammar was the minister of Trinity Episcopal Church during Wade Hampton Frost's boyhood. The Frost family always sat in a pew on the right side of the church. Years later, the following doggerel verse was found scratched into the back of the pew just in front of where the Frosts usually sat:

> Mr. Grammar is tall and slim
> His voice is grim and harsh
> He looks like a squirrel on a hickory limb
> And sounds like a frog in a marsh[23]

Local historians and long-term residents attribute this delightful mischief to Wade Hampton Frost, perhaps assisted by his brother, Tom.

Winters often brought snow storms, and the boys of Marshall turned out to go sledding on Stephenson's Hill west of town. Spring brought rain and with it mud, which bogged down carts and buggies traveling through the town. One long-time resident recalls mud so tenacious that it pulled the boots off one's feet.[24]

Frost's best friend and contemporary was John T. Ramey, son of the proprietor of one of Marshall's general stores and father of Mary Cunningham. The two boys were nearly inseparable. As they grew into adolescence, they became part of a large circle of young people from Marshall and The Plains who socialized together. Frost, strongly resembling his father, was tall, slim, and handsome. He was popular among his peers and developed a local reputation as a "party boy." At the same time, the young man was also developing more serious interests. Letters written much later suggest that he and his father, whom he called "Papa," were close, and it is likely that he was already thinking of following his father and his older brother, Henry Pinckney, into medicine. As a young boy and also during a teen-age year at home, he accompanied his father in the buggy on his daily rounds of house calls.[25] Frost's interest in a medical career developed early.

If Frost were to obtain a university education and study medicine, as his parents hoped, then schooling beyond that provided in his mother's classes would be necessary to prepare him for higher education. In the fall of 1895 the fifteen year-old Frost entered the Danville Military Institute in Danville, Virginia. A smaller school than some contemporary institutions, it provided both classical education and military training. Frost was initially somewhat homesick and felt out of place, his conservative and church-oriented upbringing setting him apart from many of his classmates. In a letter to John Ramey's mother he wrote:

> Col. Saunders got all the boarders to sign a pledge not to take any intoxicating liquor between now and the end of the session. I am very glad he did it for some of the boys would always be getting drunk. . . . I wish I could spend Sundays away from here, for the boys cut up so that I have to stay in my room unless I want to join them, and I get awfully lonesome.[26]

As one might expect, life at the school was regimented. Students were allowed to leave the campus only with written permission or to attend church. Card playing was forbidden.

Yet Frost's letters reveal that he adapted well and came to enjoy the school. He found the military drill exciting. "I think the drilling is splendid training for the mind as well as the body. It teaches you to be quick and to pay attention."[27] Frost did well in his studies. He made friends with some of his class-mates who lived in Danville, and this led to invitations to their homes. He took dancing lessons, and found himself a bit cha-grined at enjoying them. He wrote to John Ramey:

> I must say I can't see the harm in dancing once in a while. . . . You don't know how much less awkward dancing has made me. The girls who [attend the dancing school] are, for the most part, as nice as they can be. Naturally some of them are fast, but that is not the case everywhere.[28]

As is apparent from this passage, the teen-aged Frost was becoming increasingly interested in girls. Sadie Harvie, the fif-teen year-old sister of one of Frost's schoolmates, particularly attracted him. "She is a nice girl," Frost wrote to his friend, "and the boys here think she and I have quite a case, but that is hardly so."[29]

After the year in Danville, Frost, attended Randolph-Macon College for one year. Thereafter, now seventeen, he returned to Marshall for one year before enrolling in the University of Virginia. In Marshall he worked at the general store operated by the Ramey family. A letter written to John Ramey, who was still away from Marshall at a boarding school, reveals a happy youth. Much of the content of the letter concerned girls, "but" he explained, "I thought that subject would interest you more than anything else." He reported on Janie Mason, a favorite of both Frost and his friend (she later married John Ramey). Janie Beverley also caught his eye at that time. Driving horse and buggy, Frost traveled back and forth the six miles between Marshall and The Plains, where many of his friends lived, and he described some of these happy sorties to his correspondent.

> We sat around and talked awhile about "old times," "first impres-sions," etc. I got Janie [Mason] to playing and I tell you what. She is a splendid performer on the piano. That makes a very big difference with me, for I love music with all my heart.[30]

In talking about his work at the store, Frost reported that he had sold his friend's old overall jacket for twenty-five cents, which seemed to him a fair price. John's father, he noted, had sold "all of the rye he had on hand to Mr. Sinclair, about 150 [bushels]." E. L. Sinclair, known to all as "Bud," was the owner of a large distillery located about two miles from Marshall; he was reputed to make the best whiskey in the region.[31]

In the fall of 1898, Frost entered the University of Virginia. As we shall see, that marked a turning point in his life. He would only occasionally return to Marshall, although he kept up a lively correspondence with his father. His best friend, John Ramey, went to the University of Virginia with him, but after Ramey left the university that friendship waned, as did his relationships with other friends in Marshall and The Plains. Wade Hampton Frost was headed for a life in a larger world, a world that would challenge him, a world that would excite him, a world upon which he would have an enormous impact. Although he distanced himself from Marshall, the imprint of his boyhood and family life there—the stamp of that small Piedmont world—would never leave him.

4

Health of the People

For it is surprising how much of basic evidence
in epidemiology has been derived from well-
ordered, simple observation in the small field
encompassed by a local health officer.
                                —*Wade Hampton Frost*[1]

Eighteen-year-old Wade Hampton Frost entered the University
of Virginia in 1898. Both of his parents were well educated,
and they made efforts to secure higher education for those of
their children with an aptitude for learning. The young Frost
was interested in medicine, and the University of Virginia had
offered a medical degree from its inception. Thus, the decision
was easily made, and August of 1898 saw him depart to
Charlottesville to begin his university studies.

The University of Virginia was founded by Thomas
Jefferson, who had long been a promoter of higher education.
During his long political career he tried repeatedly to find a
way to establish a university in Virginia, success finally coming
with authorization and appropriation of fifteen thousand dollars by the Virginia legislature in 1818. Jefferson himself
designed the institution's grounds in Charlottesville, and on
March 7, 1825, the university opened with the aging former
president at its helm as rector. Jefferson lived only sixteen
more months. It is said he considered the University of Virginia
the finest of his many accomplishments in the service of his
fellow citizens. "If I had to decide between the pleasure
derived from a classical education which my father gave me
and the estate he left me," Jefferson is alleged to have said, "I
would decide in favor to the former."[2]

The handsome original buildings designed by Jefferson
in classical elegance are still in use today. They included a

dome-capped building known as the rotunda at the head of a gracious lawn; it was used for administrative offices. Flanking the lawn on its east and west sides were two parallel rows of buildings containing faculty and student apartments as well as classrooms. Behind the two rows of lawn buildings were two additional rows of similar buildings known as ranges. As the grounds have expanded in modern times, Jefferson's original buildings have retained their central position. During his first two student years, Frost lived in Room 42 East Lawn, sharing the room with his Marshall friend and classmate, John Ramey. In his third year, he lived in Room 11 West Range and during his last two years in 27 West Range; Ramey spent only two years at the university, and Frost did not have a roommate during those final three years.

From its inception the University of Virginia provided high-quality scholarship in a remarkably liberal academic environment. Jefferson recruited many of the first faculty members from abroad—five from England, only one, the professor of law, a Virginian. An observer contemporaneous with Frost described the university as

> An ideal community . . . a small republic, finding in itself all that is necessary in the way of government and the pursuit of happiness. It is democratic as far as its government is concerned. . . . There is no president, but there is a chairman of the faculty. . . .
>
> The atmosphere of this college world is ideal. Here a man's consequence is not determined by his wealth nor by his antecedents, but by his character. . . . There is absolute equality of opportunity, a thing necessary in an ideal republic, and the thing which was really demanded by the Declaration of Independence.[3]

Perhaps one should note that the "equality of opportunity" extended only to men; women were not admitted to the University of Virginia nor were they franchised in the democracy that Jefferson helped to forge.

A chronicler of the University of Virginia, who was a student in the post-Civil War years, wrote his reflections on the university after revisiting it shortly after Frost had been a student. He made particular note of the honor system, which committed students to pledge that they had not cheated on examinations. This pledge was not challenged by the faculty, but should an infraction come to light, dismissal would result. The chronicler further commented on those whom he thought would benefit most from education at the University of Virginia.

> It is the grateful son of honest purpose, studious habits, erudite mind, in a degree self-centered personality—not younger than eighteen— that feeds best at her shrine.[4]

The young but rapidly maturing Frost fit that description well.

During his first year as a university student, Frost was enrolled in the Academic Department, taking courses in English literature, history, economics, and mathematics. Beginning with his second year, he was also enrolled in the Department of Medicine, adding Latin and biology to his studies. The following year he studied comparative anatomy, and in ensuing years German and geology. Frost received the Bachelor of Arts degree on June 12, 1901, being awarded certificates in economics, history, and mathematics.[5] The medical curriculum which he had begun with his second university year, required four years of study. Courses offered at the time in the Medical Department, and that Frost almost certainly took, included chemistry, medical biology, anatomy, physiology, bacteriology, pathology, hygiene, obstetrics, surgery, materia medica (pharmacology), practice of medicine, therapeutics, diseases of the eye and ear, gynecology and abdominal surgery, and medical jurisprudence. Most medical students of the present day would recognize these courses. In fact, although largely didactic, the classroom curriculum in medicine at the University of Virginia in Frost's time was an exemplary one. However, the program was not strong in clinical experience. Frost received the Doctor of Medicine degree on June 17, 1903. In 1901, while still a student, he was appointed a Demonstrator of Pathology.

From October 1902 through January 1903, Frost served as editor-in-chief of *College Topics*, the twice-weekly student newspaper, a position reflecting both respect and social prestige among his fellow students. Although they were unsigned, it is fair to presume that he wrote the weekly lead editorials, which focused on student life and issues of importance to students. While many of them were commentaries on the current fall football season, some of Frost's efforts were more serious. A series of editorials sharply criticized the proposed appointment of Colonel George W. Miles to a chair in economics especially created for him and to the post of chairman of the faculty. Miles had never studied nor taught economics but had been the principal of St. Albans School of Radford, Virginia, a post from which he had resigned in anticipation of the appointment at the University of Virginia. He was a long-time member of the University Board of Visitors and close friend of many of its members. Seventeen of twenty-three faculty members had signed a petition formally protesting this bit of cronyism by the Board of Visitors. "It is now 'up to us' the students . . . to take some vigorous action," declared *College Topics*.[6] A "mass meeting" was called for, which took place three days later with considerable disturbance of the university's tranquility, including the shooting out of lights. Miles did have one qualification, however, which Frost and his student journalist colleagues noted:

> He is a man of nerve; for having never studied nor taught Economics he declares himself willing to take the professorship of that subject in the University after having "seriously looked into the subject during the summer." Greater nerve than this hath no man! Is not this very willingness to take the chair of a subject which he has only read-up during the summer the strongest possible proof on his unfitness for the place?[7]

Miles did not get the appointment. With a bit of whimsy to which students savoring victory felt themselves entitled, Frost and his coeditors commented:

> From the sad and unavailing martyrdom of Miles, we may learn several valuable lessons.
> First—A school in your own hand is worth more than a university in somebody else's hands.
> Second—Never count your chickens until the eggs are laid.
> Third—Put not your trust in some "friends."
> Fourth—Read TOPICS.[8]

One must not forget that Frost was a college student and as full of fun as college students have been at all times, from the era of his ancestor, "Jolly" Thomas Frost at Cambridge, to the modern times of spring breaks and tail-gate parties at football games. He was a member of Kappa Alpha fraternity, and joined in its social activities. He was also a member of O.W.L., a student society drawing its members from a group that today might be considered the socially elite. Figure 4.1 shows Frost with a group of his classmates. While the circumstances of this photograph are not known, they were certainly jovial. It is likely that the others in the picture were fraternity brothers. Frost wrote the following football pep song, to be sung to the tune of Strike Up the Band:

Give us a song, boys, for old Virginia
Root loud and strong, with all that's in you;
    Wake up the town
    At every down
With a yell—a long yell for
    Virginia.

Show them some "stunts," Virginia, in cunning,
Drop-kicks and punts, dodging and running;
    Through Tar Heel's line
    Gain every time
Break 'em up and shake 'em up,
    Virginia.

Champions are we, mighty and glorious,
Here's to the V, ever victorious;
    Here's to its wearers,
    Makers and bearers
Of your name and mighty fame,
    Virginia.[9]

Frost graduated from the University of Virginia in 1903. Figure 4.2 is a formal portrait of the young man taken at about the time of his commencement, perhaps a graduation picture. The young graduate could now write MD after his name, but he remained far removed from the clinical competence that would be expected of a doctor. As was typical of medical education of that time, his training at the University of Virginia had been

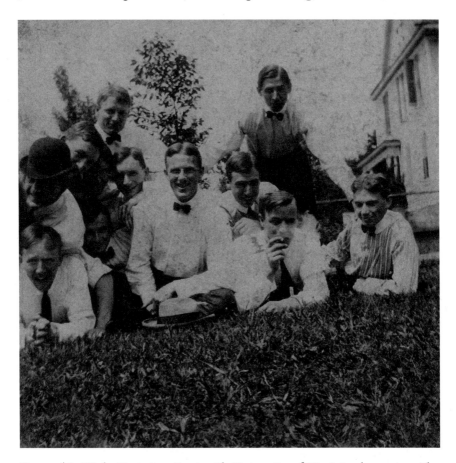

Figure 4.1. Wade Hampton Frost with University of Virginia classmates. The location is probably the lawn of the Kappa Alpha fraternity house. Frost is fourth from the right. The others are probably fraternity brothers. Photograph is from the Claude Moore Health Sciences Library, University of Virginia Health Sciences Center, Charlottesville, VA: Wade Hampton Frost Archives, Box 6, Folder 2. Reproduced with permission, courtesy of the Historical Collection and Services of the Claude Moore Health Sciences Library.

almost entirely didactic. He lacked the clinical experience necessary to develop his professional skills. Like other young medical graduates then and now he sought an internship where he could gain clinical experience under supervision while receiving further instruction. His initial selection was Bellevue Hospital in New York City. He could not have made a better choice.

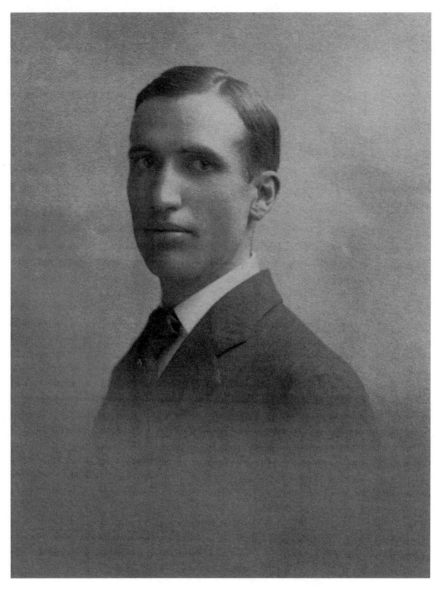

Figure 4.2. Studio photographic portrait of Wade Hampton Frost taken at about the time of his commencement from the University of Virginia. Photograph is from the Claude Moore Health Sciences Library, University of Virginia Health Sciences Center, Charlottesville, VA: Wade Hampton Frost Archives, Box 6, Folder 12. Reproduced with permission, courtesy of the Historical Collection and Services of the Claude Moore Health Sciences Library.

New York City's first hospital was the Almshouse Hospital. A medical school was established there in 1787. In 1795 it moved to the Belle Vue Farm, which the city had purchased from the Kip family. A new building was erected in 1816, and in 1825 the Bellevue name (originally Belvue) was adopted. Medical education was a prominent activity at the hospital, and additional teaching facilities were constructed during ensuing years and decades. At the time of Frost's internship, Bellevue was the clinical site for the University Medical College, which became the New York University College of Medicine in 1935.[10] The medical faculty at Bellevue was an illustrious one. Among its members was Hermann Biggs, a great pioneer of public health and director of the Carnegie Laboratory at Bellevue, the first public health laboratory in the United States.[11] Biggs was also recognized as one of the city's most skilled clinicians and was active on the teaching faculty at Bellevue. One cannot but wonder if the young Frost might not have met Biggs and been influenced in his career thinking by that preeminent sanitarian.

Frost followed his internship at Bellevue with similar experiences at St. John's Hospital in Yonkers, New York, and St. Vincent's Hospital in Norfolk, Virginia. With two years in these internships, Frost had as much or more clinical experience as any young physician of his time. He made visits to his home in Marshall from time to time during these years, and there he assisted his father on his rounds and at surgical procedures. He became known in Marshall as "the young doctor."[12] Surely there were many in Marshall, including members of his family, who hoped he would return to the town of his boyhood to take up the practice of his beloved father. But that would not happen.

During the years following graduation from the University of Virginia, Frost decided to pursue a career in public health. In a speech to the British parliament in 1877, Benjamin Disraeli had said:

> The health of the people is really the foundation upon which all their happiness and all their powers as a state depend.

Frost chose to look to the health of the people rather than the health of individual persons. He took and passed the required examinations, and on January 13, 1905, he was commissioned an Assistant Surgeon in United States Public Health Service. He was assigned to the Marine Hospital in Baltimore, Maryland, one of a system of such hospitals dating to colonial days providing medical care to seamen.

Frost's motivations in choosing a career in public health have been the subject of much speculation. Kenneth Maxcy[13] and Jack Gwaltney,[14] both themselves products of the University of Virginia, cite the strong traditions of public service among Virginia graduates. This tradition was also considered by Frost's daughter to be the principal factor in his motivation.[15] Among the public health luminaries from Virginia were Walter Reed, whose pioneering work on malaria and especially yellow fever were soon to have a direct impact on Frost's life, and Hugh Cumming, the Surgeon General during much of the time Frost served in the Public Health Service. Frost's University of Virginia graduating class of 1903 dedicated its yearbook to the memory of Reed, who had died the preceding November.[16] Cumming would become an associate and friend of Frost in subsequent years.

If his experience at the University of Virginia helped to mold Frost's altruistic career decisions, so also must have his family background—and even his name. His parents devoted their lives in Marshall to community service. His father served not only as the town's physician but also as an elder and leading figure in his church. No one was surprised when Marshall chose to name a street for Dr. Henry Frost. His mother stepped in to organize a school when it became apparent that the existing school was inadequate. A Frost family tradition of service extended back for generations, including the lives of Reverend Thomas Frost and Dr. Henry Rutledge Frost in Charleston, South Carolina. And Henry Frost was proud of his Confederate military service under General Wade Hampton (an initially reluctant but then thoroughly committed soldier)—proud enough to name a son for that great leader.

The early twentieth century was an exciting time in the world of infectious diseases. Robert Koch had unraveled the causes of first anthrax and then tuberculosis and cholera, establishing many of the fundamental techniques of bacteriology. Antiserum treatment of such diseases as diphtheria had recently arrived in dramatic fashion; the Iditarod race today commemorates a 1925 life-saving dog-sled race to Nome, Alaska, carrying the vital antiserum. Under the leadership of such men as Hermann Biggs, New York City and especially Bellevue Hospital were in the vanguard of this advancing science that for the first time in history offered hope of cure of disease. Biggs was an evangelist in the cause of public health, proclaiming to all that a community could determine the state of well-being of its citizens.[17] Surely Frost must have felt the excitement of a career in this rapidly advancing field. And at Bellevue he must have met men who could provide stimulating role models for such a career.

But before one accepts altruism as the major motivating force behind Frost's decision, there are additional questions that must be addressed. Although rapidly expanding and gaining stature, the United States Public Health Service was still at an embryonic stage of its development in 1903 and 1904, when Frost must have made his career choice. Its antecedents lay with quarantine measures enacted by the young American congress in 1799. A fiat from Surgeon General John M. Woodworth in 1875 expanded the duties of the Marine Hospital Service to include enforcement of quarantine and public health measures; in 1878 Congress passed legislation to a similar effect. In 1872, officers of the Marine Hospital Service were instrumental in organizing the American Public Health Association. A major yellow fever outbreak in the Mississippi River valley in 1877 saw the first involvement of Marine Hospital Service medical officers in a public health campaign. A National Board of Health was created in 1879, but it was of short duration and had little impact. In 1883 the Marine Hospital Service was given statutory authority over United States quarantine activities. It was the Spanish American War of 1898 with its attendant scourges of malaria and yellow fever that finally aroused public attention to issues of public health. In 1902 the Marine Hospital Service was renamed the Public Health and Marine Hospital Service, reflecting not a new but an expanded mission.[18] Thus Frost, who had entered the University of Virginia in 1898 and was a medical student in 1902, was present at the birth of the modern institution.

The great pioneers of public health in America—William Sedgwick in Boston and Hermann Biggs and T. Mitchell Prudden in New York—were not public health service officers. In fact, Sedgwick, whom many consider the first American sanitarian, was a sanitary engineer with no formal medical training. Biggs and Prudden were physicians, pathologists, and students of the new science of bacteriology. Much of the exciting field work of public health at that time, including the Walter Reed's and William Gorgas's dramatic conquest of yellow fever in Cuba, was being accomplished under the leadership of army officers. One must wonder why Frost did not choose a military career if he wanted a life of national service and public health. When he made his decision he must have anticipated assignments to Marine Hospitals, perhaps with opportunities in bacteriology and the study of infectious diseases. Realistically, a career in epidemiology could hardly have been expected by a young, newly enlisted Public Health and Marine Hospital Service officer in 1905.

There is yet another possible motive for Frost's decision that should be considered. It was raised speculatively by Phillip Sartwell, one of Frost's later colleagues, in reflecting on Frost's career.

> I believe he got tuberculosis some time during his educational career or before. . . . My suspicion is that after this he went looking for a position which would perhaps be less physically demanding. Now this is just a surmise, . . . a guess . . . , but my suspicion would be that his physicians probably told him, you can't do general practice—his father had been a physician—you can't do general practice, your constitution won't stand it, and you'd better look for something physically easier, which might have attracted him to the Public Health Service.[19]

Sartwell's surmises are merely speculation, for he had no first-hand knowledge of the events nor did he know Frost at that time. However, some degree of credence to the idea is given by Eva Anderson, the family cook who knew Frost and his family intimately. In an interview she termed Frost's 1918 episode of tuberculosis as a "break down," implying that it was not the first episode of this illness.[20] One can wonder if the year at home after leaving Randolph-Macon College and before entering the University of Virginia was intended as a period of recuperation from tuberculosis, the disease which had stricken the Frost family so frequently. As we will see, however, Frost's career in public health was hardly set at the relaxed pace one might have expected had he had major concerns about the physical limitations that medical thinking of that day imposed upon those who had suffered from tuberculosis.

Frost took up his clinical post at the Baltimore Marine Hospital, but his tenure there was urgently and dramatically interrupted after little more than a year. This interruption would introduce Frost to the excitement of field epidemiology. It would have a major impact on the young physician. It would introduce him in a meaningful way to public health and the potential accomplishments of that field. Once involved in that arena, Frost would never again focus on the care of sick individuals; he would devote his efforts to healing communities and populations of people.

It began with a telegram sent by Public Health and Marine Hospital Service Surgeon A. C. White in New Orleans, Louisiana, to the Washington headquarters of the service on July 18, 1906: "Rumors of yellow fever in New Orleans. Can learn nothing definite. Letter follows."[21]

Yellow fever is a terrible disease, caused by a virus, frequently fatal, and in its day evoking the same type of fear that Ebola virus infections do today. Like Ebola disease, it causes massive bleeding, and patients usually become deeply jaundiced before dying, which gives rise to its name. Whether it originated in Africa, the Caribbean region, or Central America is not known. The first outbreak that can clearly be identified as yellow fever occurred in the Yucatan Peninsula in 1648. The causative virus is carried by mosquitos, and the most important event in the early history of yellow fever in the Americas was the importation of *Aëdes aegypti,* the only species of mosquito that transmits this infection. This mosquito has a unique life style that facilitates transmission of the malevolent virus to people and also points the way to control efforts. This mosquito lives around people. It breeds by laying its eggs in small reservoirs of water such as cisterns, gutters, and old cans or pots. It bites in the evening and at night— rarely during the day. It does not travel far after biting an infected person, so it usually passes the virus on to someone near at hand. As this mosquito spread across the globe, so also spread yellow fever, and by the mid-nineteenth century the disease was a prevalent scourge of much of the Caribbean and Central America. It effectively prevented a French company from constructing a canal across the Panamanian isthmus during the 1880s.[22]

The conquest of yellow fever is one of the great stories of public health. Its heroes were James Carroll, Walter Reed, and William Gorgas. As early as 1881, Carlos Finlay in Cuba had suggested that yellow fever might be transmitted by mosquitoes. In 1897 Ronald Ross demonstrated that mosquitoes carried malarial parasites, a discovery for which he received the Nobel Prize in Medicine or Physiology in 1902. Carroll noted the similarity between the epidemiology of yellow fever in two outbreaks in Mississippi and that of malaria. His observations put the earlier hypothesis of Finlay on firm ground and convinced the public health community that its efforts should be directed toward the ubiquitous mosquito.[23] Gorgas was an army medical officer who himself had survived yellow fever while stationed in Texas. He was sent to Cuba in 1898 following the Spanish-American War to institute sanitary measures in the disease-ridden city of Havana.[24] Yellow fever raged, and a special commission headed by Reed was soon dispatched to Cuba. With Carroll as one of its members, the commission quickly embraced the mosquito as the vector of the virus, and Reed identified *A. aegypti* as the villain. Mosquito control began in earnest, with control of the disease the happy result of the effort. Later, Gorgas would lead the mosquito control campaign in Panama that made the successful construction of the Panama Canal possible.

New Orleans, a port city serving the endemic regions of Central and South America and the Caribbean, was continually at risk for the importation of yellow fever. An outbreak had occurred in that city in 1899 with 115 cases and twenty deaths.[25] Since that year the Louisiana city had been free of the disease. White's telegram was a wake-up call. In his letter, which arrived on July 24, 1906, White reported:

> In the forenoon of Tuesday, July 18, I was informed that there were rumors of the existence of yellow fever in a block bounded by Decatur, Charles, Ursulines, and St. Philip Streets, and that there had been deaths. I visited the region in the afternoon, and on one door saw a death notice. A woman standing by volunteered information about the character of the man's sickness and the mode of death, which made the case look very much like yellow fever.[26]

White then described a series of fruitless encounters with local physicians and health authorities who were hesitant to admit the presence of the disease in their city and reluctant to institute control measures. The attitude of the citizens of New Orleans changed from denial to alarm, however, as new cases continued to appear and it soon became apparent that a major yellow fever epidemic had struck. By August 3, 308 cases had been reported with fifty-nine deaths. On August 4, President Theodore Roosevelt directed the Public Health Service to take charge, and on August 7, 1906, eleven officers were dispatched to New Orleans, including Wade Hampton Frost.[27]

What could these sanitarians do? They could quarantine ships arriving from endemic areas as well as transports leaving the city, which might carry the pestilence elsewhere. They could place persons ill with yellow fever under netting so that they would not be bitten by mosquitoes. They could fumigate buildings. Most importantly, they could eliminate or cover with fine screening or oil the fresh-water breeding places of *A. aegypti*, not a trivial task in a city with some seven thousand cisterns. But they did it, working hard, day after day. Still, the epidemic continued with what must have been discouragingly mounting case numbers. By September 20, there had been 2,678 cases and 349 deaths. Control efforts continued, and on October 8 came the first drop in the daily tally. There were no further increases in this much-watched figure, and on November 1 the first day with no new cases arrived. Four new cases occurred during the following week, and then it was over. The final totals: 3,389 cases and 459 deaths.[28]

The achievement of Frost and the other public health officers working in New Orleans was remarkable. This was the first yellow fever epidemic aborted in the United States before the onset of a winter frost reduced the mosquito population. No one could ever again doubt the efficacy of mosquito control as a public health measure. In fact, no subsequent epidemics of yellow fever have occurred in the United States.

Frost was a changed person. What an epiphany, what a thrilling experience the New Orleans assignment must have been for Frost. Soon, he would join the growing ranks of health professionals committed not just to the sanitation aspects of public health but to the expanding field of epidemiology and its role in protecting the health of the public. Ultimately he would lead and train many of them.

Frost returned to his assigned station in Baltimore and to the care of seamen at the Marine Hospital in that city. Work at that facility was interrupted from time to time by other assignments. He spent a month screening immigrants at Ellis Island. He served from time to time as the medical officer for Coast Guard cadets in training.[29]

Summer duty for medical officers of the Public Health and Marine Hospital Service included tours aboard revenue cutters, the predecessors of today's United States Coast Guard cutters (the Public Health Service still provides medical officers for Coast Guard vessels). Frost served on the U.S.S. Chase in the summer of 1907. Figure 4.3 shows him with other officers on that vessel. The sea duty that year included a stop in Algiers. In the summer of 1908 he served on the U.S.S. Itaska, calling at Le Havre, France, among other ports. A postal card sent from Le Havre to his favorite sister, Hallie, noted that the ship

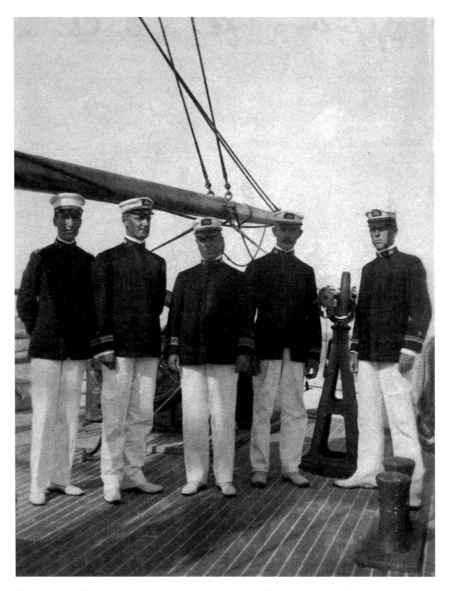

Figure 4.3. Wade Hampton Frost with other officers aboard the revenue cutter U.S.S. Chase. Frost is at the far left. Photograph is from the Claude Moore Health Sciences Library, University of Virginia Health Sciences Center, Charlottesville, VA: Wade Hampton Frost Archives, Box 6, Folder 15. Reproduced with permission, courtesy of the Historical Collection and Services of the Claude Moore Health Sciences Library.

had arrived the previous day and was now "besieged by peddlers."[30] He visited Paris on leave from his vessel at that time. Other assignments with the Coast Guard included visits to the Azores, to Spain, and to Italy. Frost was happy as a young public health officer, and he enjoyed the various tours that interrupted his medical duties.

5

Drink No Longer Water

> The opportunities for exposure . . . would
> depend largely upon proximity of dwellings,
> customs with respect to excreta disposal, and
> character of food and source of drinking water.
> —*Wade Hampton Frost*[1]

Without water, life would not exist on earth. Without drinking water, humans cannot survive. Without safe drinking water, people cannot remain disease-free. Harmful parasites, bacteria, and viruses all inhabit fresh water, and if we are to have safe drinking water, they must be killed or removed. The New Testament enjoins, "Drink no longer water, but use a little wine for thy stomach's sake and thine often infirmities."[2] Today, we all assume that municipal water delivered into our homes is safe to drink. It was not always so.

Massachusetts established a state hygienic laboratory in 1886, and William T. Sedgwick, perhaps the first of America's great sanitarians, was the state bacteriologist at that facility. Sedgwick identified the town's contaminated drinking water as the cause of a typhoid fever outbreak in Lowell, Massachusetts, and this led to the construction in that community of the first North American municipal water filtration plant. Although chlorination of water, the technique most widely used today to render water free of disease-producing microorganisms, had been used for some time in Europe, it was not introduced into North American water supply systems until 1908 when it was first applied in Jersey City, New Jersey.[3] Even today, although safe drinking water is widely available to them, many North Americans and Europeans buy bottled drinking water at prices exceeding what they pay for gasoline.

The recognition that specific microorganisms cause disease emerged in Europe with the dawning of the Renaissance, although smallpox and plague were already well known—even earlier in Asia—and were widely recognized as contagious by the general public, if not by physicians. Hieronymus Frascatorius of Verona is often cited as the first European to argue for the infectious nature of many diseases. His 1584 list of contagious ailments included "scabies, phthisis, itch, baldness, elephantiasis, and others of this sort."[4] In 1683, Antonj van Leeuwenhoek used one of his primitive, simple microscopes to examine the "scurf" of his teeth and, to his "great surprise perceived . . . many small Animals, which moved themselves very extravagantly."[5] One can identify bacteria commonly found in the mouth from Leeuwenhoek's drawings. In 1699 the Republic of Lucca in Italy enacted the first quarantine laws; at that time the concept of disease contagion was still foreign to mainstream medical thought in Northern Europe. In 1720 Benjamin Marten, an English physician, argued that tuberculosis as well as "itch, leprosy, and venereal distemper" were caused by the small organisms seen by Leeuwenhoek.[6] Proof of the transmissibility of infections was finally provided in 1767 by the tragic experiment of John Hunter, who inoculated himself with gonorrheal pus and at the same time inadvertently infected himself with syphilis, which ultimately caused his death.[7]

Proof that an identifiable microorganism caused a specific disease came with the work of Louis Pasteur, who established with a series of studies conducted during the 1860s that pebrine, a disease of silkworms, was caused by a microsporidial parasite that had first been observed in 1837 by Agostino Maria Bassi. With respect to bacterial causes of human disease, credit for discovery belongs to that unparalleled giant of medical history, Robert Koch, who demonstrated the life cycle of the anthrax bacillus in 1876 and the etiologic role of the tubercle bacillus in 1882.[8] After his work, no doubt could remain that the microbial world contained enemies against which humans needed to protect themselves.

And what of water, that sustainer of life? There are many diseases—some caused by parasites, some by bacteria, some by viruses—that are transmitted by drinking water, especially water contaminated by sewage. Among them is typhoid fever, now no longer a problem because drinking water is treated to kill the bacterium that causes it, along with other dangerous microorganisms. Immunization is available to those who must travel or live in areas where drinking water is not safe. However, Henry Frost knew typhoid; he referred to it in a letter to his son as late as 1913:

> I think there is very little typhoid fever about. I have given anti-typhoid vaccine to several; it is quite a fad here now, and readily obtained since the State furnishes it for 90 cts (in syringes) for the three doses.[9]

Typhoid was still a prevalent and dangerous disease as Wade Hampton Frost entered upon his career.

In 1874 William Budd published a remarkable monograph entitled "Typhoid Fever. Its Nature, Mode of Spreading, and Prevention."[10] It followed earlier reports in the British medical journal, *Lancet*, in 1857, one an anonymous editorial and the second a description by Budd of an outbreak of typhoid at an orphanage, with clear identification of feces as the source of transmission of the disease.[11] Wade Hampton Frost read this work as a young physician embarking on a career in public health, and it had a major impact upon him. It was, in his mind, a paragon of epidemiologic investigation.

Budd was born in North Tawton, Devonshire, England, in 1811, one of ten children of Samuel and Catherine Budd. Samuel Budd was a surgeon, and six of his sons became doctors. William Budd studied medicine in Paris, at Middlesex Hospital in London, and in Edinburgh. His studies were interrupted by a prolonged bout of typhoid. He went on to become one of the most distinguished physicians in Britain of his era. He is remembered today as a great pioneer of epidemiology.

At the time of Budd's exposition on typhoid, a bacterial causation had not been established for any disease, and, as noted, concepts of contagion were not universally accepted. Typhoid was a disease of immense importance. Budd estimated that about 140,000 cases occurred each year in Great Britain and that the mortality rate was about ten percent of those afflicted. Budd carefully described a number of outbreaks of typhoid, noting in each case that the center of the outbreak was a privy, sewer, or other means of the disposal of feces. In many cases, these facilities were grossly offensive, but outbreaks of typhoid did not occur until a patient with the disease began to use the common facility. Moreover, isolation of typhoid patients was ineffective if the patients' feces were disposed of in common with those of others. Budd noted that fecal contamination of drinking water was a common element, but he also believed—incorrectly, as we know today—that there was airborne transmission of the causative agent from sewage. He conceived of typhoid as a sort of smallpox of the intestine with lesions in the gut similar to the skin lesions of smallpox. Since it was clear to him that smallpox was transmitted through the air, he erroneously supposed the same would be true of typhoid.

The work of Budd has been repeatedly cited as one of the great landmarks of field epidemiology. It stands as an exemplar of outbreak investigation, of "shoe leather epidemiology," of careful and detailed study of the disease and its victims in their environment. Detailed descriptions of patients, careful consideration of the time course of the outbreaks, and meticulous study of the environment including sewage and water systems characterized Budd's reports. He described many incidents of apparent transmission of typhoid fever that provided convincing evidence for the infectious nature of this disease. He went on to examine four outbreaks in detail, and in each case he considered that contamination of drinking water by sewage represented the major mode of transmission.

Let us consider Budd's discussion of the 1839 outbreak in North Tawton, Devonshire, which he characterized as the "most memorable" of the several outbreaks he reported. One case occurring in a family was usually followed by other cases in the same family. Budd carefully described the spread of disease within families. Work places were focal points for the spread of the outbreak, and travelers appeared to spread the epidemic. There could be little doubt of the contagiousness of typhoid fever. Budd addressed the mode of spread of typhoid in North Tawton. He recognized the importance of fecal transmission:

> [Outbreaks of typhoid] never occur except under one condition—that is to say, where no sufficient provisions have been made for preventing the discharges from the human intestine from contaminating the soil and air of the inhabited area. Where these provision are wanting, the most spacious rooms, and the freest internal ventilation, afford no security against the spread of the fever.[12]

Each dwelling in North Tawton, or sometimes each group of dwellings, was served by a privy. In these privies, Budd noted, "discharges continue to accumulate, day by day." Ultimately, he concluded, persons are infected when disease agents "distill . . . slowly into the water they drink."[13] As we shall see, Budd's classic work was to presage impressive field studies of typhoid by Wade Hampton Frost.

Budd's work did not stand in lonely isolation, either as an indictment of contaminated water or as a model of epidemiological investigation. In 1849 in preliminary fashion and more definitively in 1855 John Snow published a monograph entitled "On the Mode of Communication of Cholera."[14] Snow was a London physician and surgeon who had first met cholera during an outbreak in Newcastle in 1831 and 1832. Cholera had been endemic since antiquity in the large river deltas of the Indian subcontinent. Snow noted that it first afflicted British troops serving in that area in 1814 and within a decade had begun to spread globally, often traveling with afflicted passengers on ships. The first case in London occurred in a newly arrived British seaman in 1848; an epidemic followed during the ensuing year. In what Wade Hampton Frost called "a nearly perfect model" in his introduction to the republished edition of the work, Snow carefully analyzed the distribution of cholera in London looking for factors that might explain its clustering. He soon focused on water supplies and demonstrated that cholera occurred more than three times more frequently in houses served by the Southwark and Vauxhall Water Works than in houses served by other water companies. Snow focused particular attention on a water pump in Broad Street, from which the handle was ultimately removed as part of the efforts to control the epidemic.

Snow's work differed from that of Budd. While the latter concentrated on careful examination of diseased individuals and their environs, Snow looked at a large body of incidence data. Frost became familiar with the work of both of these pioneers. In his career, he would use both of their approaches, and he would use their studies in his teaching. His early investigations of disease outbreaks, as a public health service officer, drew inspiration from the painstaking attention to detail and meticulous data collection of Budd. As his career evolved, Frost would make major contributions in the analysis of large sets of epidemiologic data of the type collected by Snow. Frost, who greatly admired both of these pioneer epidemiologists, would follow in their footsteps and broaden the trail for those who were to follow. In doing so, he would bring to North America a germinating scientific discipline, the prior seeds of which had all brought forth rudimentary sprouts in Europe.

Thus it was that the science of epidemiology was born, ushered into the world by the nineteenth-century midwifery of John Snow and William Budd. Their studies of two important waterborne illnesses preceded the identification of the actual causative agents. *Salmonella typhi*, the cause of typhoid fever, was isolated in 1880 by Georg Gaffkey working at the Koch Institute in Berlin. *Vibrio cholera*, the microorganism that causes cholera, was first isolated by Robert Koch in India in 1884.

As the twentieth century dawned, the United States reveled in rapidly advancing technology. Railroads, electric lights, automobiles, assembly lines, even flying machines—what was there that the modern age could not accomplish? Meanwhile, medical scientists—Koch, Pasteur, and their colleagues in Europe and also Theobald Smith, William Welch, and others in North America—were identifying an increasing number of microorganisms that caused disease. Surely the time was ripe for this new knowledge to be applied to public health. Surely the public could be protected from typhoid fever, cholera, and other diseases.

The earliest legislative attempts to promote public health in America date to the colonial era. During the reign of George III, seamen sailing in and out of American ports were taxed to support the medical care of British sailors at the Royal Hospital in Greenwich, England. In 1768 the Federal Marine Hospital Service in the American colonies was established by charter from the king, and that organization is now looked upon as the earliest progenitor of the United States Public Health Service. In the mid-eighteenth century laws regulating medical practice were enacted in Virginia, Massachusetts, New York, and New Jersey. In 1796 the first national law of the United States relevant to public health provided for the use of revenue cutters and military facilities to assist states in enforcing their quarantine and health laws. In 1797 the Fifth Congress of the United States imposed a tax of twenty cents on every seaman on every vessel docking in the ports of the new United States to support medical care for American seamen.[15]

As medical knowledge advanced during the nineteenth century, the health of the public was increasingly viewed as of civic concern, and by 1900, forty states had established health departments. At that time the leading causes of death in the United States were pneumonia, tuberculosis, and diarrhea and enteritis, in that order. Heart disease and other ailments that lead the list today followed.[16] Clearly, things could be done about those leading killers. As Hermann Biggs, a pioneer public health commissioner of New York, repeatedly said, "public health is purchasable."[17]

In August 1887 Joseph J. Kinyoun, a Marine Hospital Service physician who had studied with some of the great microbiologists of Europe, opened a bacteriology laboratory at the Marine Hospital on Staten Island, New York. There he studied cholera and other diseases afflicting persons arriving in New York aboard ships. This laboratory was the progenitor of the Public Health Service laboratories that would ultimately evolve into the National Institutes of Health. It was moved to Washington in 1891 when Walter Wyman, the director of the Staten Island hospital, became Surgeon General of the Public Health Service. Kinyoun returned to Europe, studying at the Pasteur Institute and making substantial contributions to the techniques used in the preparation of diphtheria antiserum. In 1899 Kinyoun yielded his post to Harvard-trained Milton J. Rosenau, who had joined the Marine Hospital Service in 1890.[18] Rosenau remained director of the laboratory until 1909, at which time he returned to Harvard to join the faculty of its medical school. Congress acted in March 1901 to establish the Hygienic Laboratory of the Public Health Service in Washington. Incorporating Rosenau's Marine Hospital Laboratory, it was charged with the "investigation of infectious and contagious diseases and matters pertaining to the public health."[19] This act included an appropriation of thirty-five thousand dollars, which allowed the laboratory to build a new facility on a five-acre site on Twenty-fifth Street Northwest. In 1902 the Marine Hospital Service, of which the laboratory was a dependant unit, was renamed the Public Health and Marine Hospital Service. At the same time its mandate was broadened to include the collection and publication of vital statistics. Soon thereafter the service became simply the United States Public Health Service.

Now in new and expanded facilities, the Hygienic Laboratory chose to embark on studies of the safety of drinking water, but its resources were limited and its initial efforts were limited to the investigation of outbreaks, especially of typhoid fever. The Potomac River came under early study, as would be expected given the site of the laboratory in Washington. Between 1910 and 1912 the water pollution efforts of the Public Health Service were extended to include the Great Lakes and the major rivers of the central parts of the country. Waterborne diseases were of great concern in the United States, as they were elsewhere in Europe and North America. Among them, typhoid fever was perhaps the most feared. In 1908, the year Frost joined the staff of the Hygienic Laboratory, the national death rate from typhoid fever was 25.3 per 100,000 persons; in Washington, D.C. it was 39.4; in Columbus, Ohio 110.5.[20]

In the autumn of 1908 Frost was assigned to the Hygienic Laboratory in Washington. This assignment was a "plum" given to only a few outstanding officers of the Public Health Service. Somehow, perhaps from his work during the New Orleans yellow fever outbreak, Frost became known to Rosenau who managed to arrange the assignment. In 1975 Ernest Stebbins, one of Frost's students, who later became dean of the Johns Hopkins School of Hygiene and Public Health, reflected on this assignment.

> He was one of the most active of that group of "young Turks," you'd call them, in the Public Health Service. . . . Probably Rosenau and . . . some of the more senior people at the Hygienic Laboratory may have heard about Frost or may have had some contact with him when he was working on yellow fever and felt, "here's a bright man, let's bring him in."[21]

The laboratory staff was not large. In the Division of Pathology and Bacteriology headed by Rosenau, to which Frost was assigned, there were only six officers in addition to Rosenau. The roster included John F. Anderson, Leslie L. Lumsden, Charles Vogel, Herbert M. Manning, W. W. Miller, and Lasher Hart.[22] They were a group of dedicated, competent investigators, and established for themselves a climate of imaginative and critical thought. Anderson and Lumsden, in particular, would play important roles in Frost's career.

At that time Frost had had no laboratory experience, but he plunged into his duties and quickly mastered the techniques of microbiological research. He was assigned to work on three ongoing studies that would familiarize him with the work of the laboratory and with techniques currently used for the study of transmissible diseases. These more-or-less simultaneously conducted investigations included studies of drinking water pollution, including typhoid fever, of polio, and of anaphylaxis (a term now used specifically to describe a severe, often fatal allergic reaction with shock and constriction of the airway but used more generally at that time to include many aspects of antibody-mediated allergic reactions). In these studies he worked together with others of the laboratory staff, acquiring not only their bench techniques and practical "know-how," but also learning what they knew of the nature of the relevant diseases. This mentor-student educational model would become the one in which he would later excel as a professor of epidemiology.

Among other investigative activities, Frost was assigned to work on the bacteria present in drinking water taken from the Potomac River. In fact, typhoid fever was a subject of major interest to Rosenau, who had recently conducted extensive studies of the disease in Washington and concluded that contaminated milk was the major source of typhoid transmission in that city.[23] Rosenau may have had some reason to believe that the river should be further investigated and delegated the matter of water contamination to Frost. This project may have been given to him as a method of acquainting him with the bacteriologic techniques then in use in the laboratory.

Rosenau left the Hygienic Laboratory only a year later to assume a Harvard professorship. John F. Anderson then assumed the directorship, and Frost and Leslie L. Lumsden became the lead investigators of the bacterial contamination of water. Lumsden was older than Frost, a seasoned field investigator with an established reputation in typhoid. Frost admired him and learned much from him. Lumsden was also an eccentric:

> It [was] said that when he was on an assignment to do a study of an epidemic he would drink a quart of whiskey a day, but still just be as alert and keen as he could be.[24]

What Frost had to learn how to do, with proficiency, was to sample and culture water collected from many sources. Using a sterile pipette and taking care to avoid any contamination, he removed carefully measured aliquots of water from each sample and placed them on bacteriologic culture plates and in tubes of culture medium. After incubation to allow bacterial growth, he then picked individual colonies of bacteria from the culture plates using a sterilized small wire loop and streaked them on new plates, where they were allowed to grow. Then, by studying their morphology and performing appropriate chemical tests, he identified each of the bacteria he had isolated from the water. Some strains were also injected into guinea pigs to see if they produced disease in these animals. Finally, using techniques he learned in his studies of anaphylaxis, he studied the reactions of antiserum to typhoid with the organisms he isolated. None of these techniques were exotic at the time.

From Robert Koch to William Welch, they had been developed and put into practice by many early bacteriologists. But they were new to Frost.

Frost's diligence and aptitude did not go unnoticed. On February 9, 1909, he was promoted from Assistant Surgeon to Passed Assistant Surgeon.

In October 1909 Frost presented a paper to the American Public Health Association annual meeting describing a bacterium he had isolated from Washington's drinking water; it was published a year later as a brief report, his first scientific publication.[25] He concluded that this organism was related to the typhoid bacillus, but not the cause of typhoid itself. By February of 1910 Frost had identified the organism as *Pseudomonas protea*, and he submitted a detailed report of his studies, which was published in the Hygienic Laboratory Bulletin.[26] He reported that he had made 107 cultures from sixty-seven drinking water samples collected in Washington between August 7 and December 31, 1909. Nine water samples yielded the organism.

Frost's report was remarkable not only for the large body of data he collected in a short time but also for the care with which he analyzed and discussed the results of this, his first, investigation. While the paper reveals that Frost had mastered the basic bacteriologic techniques of the laboratory, an epidemiologic perspective is evident in this early work. He investigated various types of water in the Washington area, as well as the municipal tap water. He noted that the organism was not present in raw, unfiltered water and considered various possible reasons for this observation—not solely the obvious one that the bacterium might have been introduced during filtration. Frost then went on to discuss the relationships between proteus and typhoid organisms. Clearly Frost had become familiar with and understood the relevant prior literature on the bacteriology of water and typhoid fever. Although he did not cite Budd's work in his bibliography, there can be little doubt that he knew it well at that time. In 1911 Frost presented a further report on the bacteriology of the Potomac River.[27] As before, typhoid germs were not found, but related bacilli were.

While Frost was studying drinking water taken from the Potomac River, a typhoid outbreak was underway in the southwestern West Virginia town of Williamson. Recognizing that typhoid may be a waterborne disease, the town had voted to issue bonds to provide funds to improve its public water supply. Advice was sought from the West Virginia State Board of Health, which in turn asked for help from the Surgeon General of the U.S. Public Health Service. Frost, now with only slightly more than a year's experience in studying polluted water, was assigned the task, and in May 1910 he arrived in Williamson. This type of assignment was fairly routine for the laboratory staff. However, Frost did not approach the task as routine. His report is an elegant exposition of the power of field epidemiology.[28] Moreover, Frost's investigation provided a second major epiphany for him. New Orleans had introduced him to public health and led to his laboratory assignment. Williamson would alter his course again. He stepped away from the laboratory bench. He would not be a bacteriologist, although he would not forget the important role of bacteriology in unraveling the puzzles of infections diseases. He would be an epidemiologist, and he would become a great pioneer in that increasingly important field.

Frost arrived in Williamson in May 1910. He met with local health officials and enlisted the help of local physicians. He considered the classical sources of typhoid infection—"the usual suspects," milk and to a lesser degree other foodstuffs, water, and direct contact with afflicted persons. However, it must have been immediately evident to him that the town's water was the source of the problem. Williamson drew its water from the Tug Fork of the Big Sandy River. Frost described this water as follows:

> The water supplied is of very displeasing appearance. . . . It is frequently too black to be fit for bathing and laundry purposes, and often has an offensive odor.[29]

A more superficial investigator might have simply identified typhoid germs in this water, which Frost did, and concluded the investigation with little ado, but Frost was not a superficial investigator. Working with great speed—he spent only three weeks in Williamson—he gathered information from local physicians about the course of the epidemic, he carefully mapped the town and all of the cases, he studied not only the town water system but several private wells, he studied the sewage systems and privies of Williamson and of settlements upstream from the town, and he examined the possible roles of sources of infection other than water.

From surveys of the town's doctors, Frost learned that typhoid was an endemic disease in the area; it was always present. In the late fall of 1909, typhoid began to appear with unusual frequency. Between November 1, 1909, and June 1, 1910, 152 individuals became ill with typhoid and eleven died of the disease. Frost estimated that that represented an incidence of 3,040 per 100,000 person per year; that is, an infection rate at which one in every thirty-three persons would become ill with typhoid each year. The cases, as plotted on a town map by Frost, occurred throughout the entire town and also the smaller community of East Williamson located upriver from Williamson. Moreover, second cases in the same household were usually sufficiently separated in time as to make direct contact unlikely. Only one dairy served the town, and its milk was pasteurized, but occasionally unpasteurized milk was sold by local farmers.

Williamson drew its water from the river through an intake caisson located near the center of the town. It was filtered through gravel, but not otherwise purified. More than eighty percent of those who had developed typhoid drank this water regularly. On the other hand, the Williamson Coal Company had a deep well serving its employees, and no individual who drank only that water became ill.

With respect to Williamson's sewage systems, Frost noted that:

> The town is at present only partially provided with a closed sewer system. . . . The main sewer terminates in an open ravine about one hundred yards distant from the river, and through this ravine empties into the Tug River about opposite the center of the town below the intake for the water supply. . . .

The Williamson Branch section of the town has no closed sewer system. Some of the houses on the lower portion of this branch have sewers which empty directly into [a] stream. . . . The remainder of the houses in this section are provided with open privies. . . . Every rain must wash a large portion of the contents of these privies . . . into the stream, which thus becomes an open sewer. . . . This stream empties into the Tug River about two hundred yards above the present intake for the town water supply and upon the same side of the river. . . .

East Williamson . . . has no sewers. The houses in this section of the town are provided with open privies. . . . The surface washings of the whole of East Williamson are carried into the river within a mile above the intake for the city water supply.[30]

Upstream from Williamson were a number of coal mines and camps. All of them were served by privies, mostly on the river bank. Since patients with typhoid excrete the causative bacillus in their feces, the problem in Williamson was evident. Frost recommended improvements in sewage treatment and water purification.

It is difficult not to note the similarities between Frost's study of Williamson and the early report of Budd. Frost followed in the footsteps of the early pioneer in carefully and thoroughly examining the setting of the outbreak and documenting its course. In this investigation Frost applied techniques that would become standard for future generations of field epidemiologists to identify the probable cause of an epidemic and to carefully exclude other possible causes. Several years later the meticulous and thorough Frost, drawing on his experience investigating water-related outbreaks of typhoid, emphasized the importance of not assuming the obvious in investigations of such epidemics:

In the case of a water supply used by a large majority of the population the mere fact that all the typhoid patients have drunk this water is obviously of no special significance, since this would necessarily be so, no matter what the cause of the epidemic. It is . . . necessary to *exclude other vehicles of infection*, to show that the water supply is the *only* vehicle of infection common to a significant portion of the cases. The next step in the evidence is to demonstrate the probability that the water supply was infected with typhoid bacilli at such a time as to account for the epidemic. . . . Finally, . . . all the other circumstances

[must] be more fully consistent with this than with any other hypothesis, forming a conclusive chain of circumstantial evidence.[31]

Frost's logic was elegant and impeccable and his conclusions unassailable. He did not simply accept the obvious; he carefully excluded all other possibilities. To this day, that degree of thoroughness is a pillar of all successful field investigations conducted by epidemiologists. Later in his career, Frost would develop new epidemiological concepts and approaches that would buttress field investigations of disease outbreaks. With the Williamson investigation, the first of his field studies, he joined his colleagues at the Hygienic Laboratory in setting for themselves and others an enduring standard of excellence in what has come to be known as "shoe leather epidemiology."

During 1910 and 1911, Frost conducted investigations of typhoid in Arkansas and Iowa. In October 1911, he published a report of his studies of the occurrence of typhoid in Fort Smith, Arkansas.[32] Drawing on data collected by local health officers to supplement the findings of his visit to the city, he noted that typhoid had been a problem there for at least the preceding decade, with death rates three to four times those in comparable American cities. "The present water supply of Fort Smith," he wrote, "must be considered objectionable both for esthetic and sanitary reasons."[33] However, only about one-third of the typhoid victims drank this water. Frost considered other sources of infection, especially including milk, and then made recommendations for water purification, control of the milk supply, sewage and garbage disposal, and continued public health surveillance. Both at Fort Smith and elsewhere Frost considered contaminated milk to be one of the most important means of transmission of typhoid and, by pasteurization, one of the most easily controlled.[34]

Typhoid and water pollution were not the only problems tackled by Frost. Bacteriology was not his only bench laboratory assignment. The nascent techniques of immunology also came within his purview.

That diphtheria could be treated with antiserum to the toxin prepared by immunizing horses was one of the major discoveries of the science of immunology emerging in Europe at the end of the nineteenth century. Emil von Behring was awarded the first Nobel Prize in Medicine or Physiology in 1901 for his role in this dramatic medical breakthrough. It was soon recognized that horse serum was not entirely benign, however, and the entities of serum sickness and acute anaphylaxis were recognized as unfortunate occasional consequences of the development of antibodies to the horse serum that carried the life-saving antitoxin antibodies. Anaphylaxis was sometimes fatal, and as methods for the quantitative study of antibodies developed they were applied to this matter. John F. Anderson was engaged in such studies at the Hygienic Laboratory, and Frost worked with him as his assistant, thus learning the immunological assay techniques of that time. In 1910, Frost joined Anderson as coauthor on a paper describing a large number of studies aimed at quantifying the antigen-antibody reactions producing anaphylaxis in guinea pigs.[35] To a modern scientific reader, these studies seem elementary and not appropriately designed to advance scientific knowledge. However, one must remember that the state of the art was primitive at that time. It is impressive that Anderson and Frost related all of their experiments to studies recently carried out in European laboratories and reported in European scientific journals, usually in German, sometimes in French. Clearly Anderson was conversant with the work of his European contemporaries, and Frost, with the classical education given to him by his mother and extended at the University of Virginia, must have joined his mentor in digging into the German and French reports.

Frost's collaboration with Anderson also included studies of polio, a much-feared disease in which Frost would maintain an interest long after leaving the Hygienic Laboratory. Indeed, Frost would make substantial contributions to our knowledge of this disease.

An ancient disease, polio first began to appear in epidemics late in the nineteenth century when better sanitation resulted in children, who usually had mild infections, reaching adulthood without immunity from unnoticed childhood disease.[36] In 1887, the first major epidemic of polio to be recognized in adults occurred in Stockholm, Sweden. Further epidemics occurred early in the twentieth century in Scandinavia, and in 1907 a major outbreak occurred in New York City. The following year there were multiple epidemics in the United States. In 1908 Karl Landsteiner and Erwin Popper in Vienna inoculated two monkeys with ground material from the spinal cord of a boy who had died of polio. Seventeen days later the monkeys developed paralysis. It was soon shown that the agent transmitting the disease passed through bacterial filters. That is, it was a virus.

In 1910 two French scientists reported that serum from the blood of a child with a mild illness considered to be abortive poliomyelitis contained protective antibodies.[37] Anderson and Frost read the French report of their work. They obtained filtered spinal cord extract from a monkey with polio from Simon Flexner at the Rockefeller Institute in New York City. As noted below, an epidemic of polio had just occurred in Iowa City, Iowa, and they prepared nine mixtures of serum from children who had mild cases without paralysis and the virus-containing filtrate. When these mixtures were injected into monkeys, the animals remained well, demonstrating that the sera of these children contained protective antibodies.[38] Interestingly, Anderson and Frost published their report not in the *Hygienic Laboratory Bulletin*, where much of the work of the laboratory appeared, but in the *Proceedings of the Society for Experimental Biology and Medicine* and the *Journal of the American Medical Association*, leading scientific and medical journals of the day. Clearly, they considered their observations important.

In September 1910 Frost attended the annual meeting of the American Public Health Association in Milwaukee, Wisconsin. Although not on the formal agenda of the meeting, outbreaks of polio were much on the minds of the members of the association, and two informal meetings were held, both attended by Frost. Consensus was reached that polio should become a reportable disease, that patients with polio should be quarantined in their homes, and that measures should be developed for the sanitary disinfection and disposal of wastes from patients.

It was Frost who took on the task of summarizing these recommendations for publication in the society's journal.[39]

Pursuing the line of thinking that polio was contagious, Anderson and Frost noted that their former colleague, Milton Rosenau, now at Harvard, had allowed stable flies *(Stomoxys calcitrans)* to bite monkeys with polio and then bite healthy monkeys. Six of the twelve monkeys thus exposed developed signs of polio. Anderson and Frost sought to confirm this observation. They inoculated a monkey with poliovirus and allowed it to be bitten by stable flies trapped in Washington. As expected, these flies transmitted polio to healthy monkeys.[40] While no more than confirmatory, this paper documents that Frost had acquired not only laboratory bench skills but also the techniques of studying disease in animals.

As emphasized by his work with typhoid, Frost was becoming increasingly interested in reaching out from the laboratory to field epidemiology. In the summer of 1909 he went to Iowa City, Iowa, to investigate an outbreak of nearly five hundred cases of polio. His investigation was a model of thoroughness. In the words of a later commentator, "he chose . . . to collect and assemble the evidence painstakingly, systematically, even tediously."[41] He visited sixty-seven houses and saw 118 cases of polio, which he classified as either paralytic (74 cases) or abortive (44 cases). Serum collected from these patients formed the basis for the studies of protective antibodies described above. Frost included this experience in a paper he presented to the Tenth Annual Conference of Sanitary Officers of New York on November 18, 1910 and published on the same date discussing the epidemiology of polio.[42] He noted that direct contagion by close contact could not explain the spread of cases, which he had carefully mapped in Iowa City. He concluded by discussing the usual control measures of isolation and disinfection and their limitations.

Iowa City was not the only site of Frost's field investigation of polio. Over a two-year period from 1910 to 1912, he investigated outbreaks in several communities in Iowa; in Cincinnati, Ohio, and neighboring Covington, Kentucky; and in Buffalo and Batavia, New York. These investigations were carried out with the same thoroughness as had been his study of typhoid in Williamson, West Virginia. Frost personally examined 473 individual with paralytic disease and reviewed the records of hundreds more. In each community, he carefully mapped the cases and plotted the times of their occurrence to document the course of the outbreak. He published his findings in a monumental report prepared in 1913, just at the end of his tenure at the Hygienic Laboratory.[43] John R. Paul, a virologist and epidemiologist who devoted much of his life to the study of poliomyelitis and who wrote a detailed and authoritative account of the history of that disease, commented on Frost's field work with polio as follows:

> Before Frost, no man had gone out into so many communities to deal with epidemic poliomyelitis with such sophisticated weapons; and, it might be added, few investigators were to use these combined approaches in epidemiological research on this disease again, for at least another twenty years.[44]

A major advance in understanding of the fundamental nature of poliomyelitis resulted from Frost's studies. Following polio epidemics in Sweden in 1887 and 1911, W. Wernstedt proposed that mild childhood infections without paralysis or other clinical illness produced lasting immunity.[45] This hypothesis was initially published in Sweden, but was later reported at a conference in Washington in 1912, which Frost almost certainly attended. As noted previously, Frost and Anderson had demonstrated antibodies to polio virus in the serum of asymptomatic children, an observation that supported this hypothesis. With his field investigations, Frost went further in advancing our understanding of this disease. He stated his conclusions elegantly in his 1913 report:

> There are certain facts which suggest that the very general immunity of adults may be specific, acquired from previous unrecognized infection with the virus of poliomyelitis. The facts which suggest this are as follows:
>
> 1. Poliomyelitis is known to occur in forms quite difficult to recognize clinically. There is, indeed, good reason to believe that

> even during epidemics the number of cases without paralysis
> exceeds the number of paralytic cases. . . . It is obvious that
> such cases, without the development of paralysis, which may
> perhaps be considered as a complication or accident, would
> never be recognized as poliomyelitis.
>
> 2. The perennial occurrence of sporadic cases shows that the
>   infection is and has been endemic . . . for a number of
>   years. . . .
> 3. The spontaneous decline of epidemics in localities where only
>   a very small percentage of the population have been attacked,
>   and the subsequent immunity of these localities while the
>   epidemic spreads in contiguous localities suggests that a pop-
>   ulation may be immunized by an epidemic giving rise to only
>   one recognized case of poliomyelitis among several hundred
>   or several thousand inhabitants. . . . [46]

Thus, carefully and meticulously, Frost marshaled the epidemiological evidence implicating mild childhood infections as
the cause of adult immunity and the change of polio from its
historical infantile paralysis form to that of the devastating adult
disease more commonly seen in modern times. This trail-
blazing concept, first introduced obscurely in Sweden during
the prior year and now stated with exceptional clarity and vigor
by Frost, is fundamental to our understanding of poliomyelitis.
Without this knowledge, the world-wide vaccination campaigns
and the necessary accompanying monitoring of viral transmission could never have been born. These global programs have
been responsible for our conquest of this crippling disease;
Frost's work created a fundamental part of the knowledge that
made that victory possible.

New York was among the first of the American states to
institute reporting of cases of polio, and in 1911 Frost published an elegant epidemiologic analysis of data collected in
New York State in 1908, 1909, and 1910.[47] He examined the
geographic location, seasonal incidence and age distribution,
and the morbidity and mortality of the disease. His conclusions
touched not only upon the epidemiology and possible control
measures, but upon such clinically relevant aspects as prognosis; Frost had not forgotten that he was a doctor. The same year
he also published a comprehensive review of polio covering

all aspects of the disease in what might serve as a text for health professionals.[48]

In June 1911 Frost reported to the annual meeting of the American Medical Association as chairman of the Committee on Methods for the Control of Poliomyelitis.[49] In the preceding year 5,093 cases with 539 deaths had been reported from thirty-one states, the District of Columbia, and Hawaii. The report reviewed the current situation of epidemic polio in the United States and made recommendations regarding diagnosis, reporting, and control measures. With respect to the latter, however, the report noted that "the committee [was] unable to express any great confidence in the efficacy of the measures . . . outlined."[50] Additional committee and conference work and reports of these activities followed.[51] Frost, now only eight years out of medical school, had rapidly become a national expert on polio and spokesperson as the nation faced the mounting challenges of this increasingly prevalent disease with its panic-inducing summer outbreaks. John Paul credits Frost's work on that disease with introducing statistical epidemiology to the study of disease in general: "To no man more than Frost is credit due for establishing epidemiology as a biological and statistical science in this country."[52]

In the spring of 1911 Frost was sent to Savannah, Georgia, to investigate an outbreak of fifty cases of meningococcal meningitis, a disastrous infection of the membranes covering the brain and spinal cord due to a bacterium now named *Neisseria meningitidis*. Meningococcal meningitis occurs sporadically and also in outbreaks or epidemics. The causative microorganism may be carried in the throats of healthy individuals. Prior to the introduction of sulfonamides and antibiotics, this disease was invariably fatal. However, antiserum containing antibodies directed against the causative bacterium was available in Frost's time, and it constituted the mainstay of treatment for this infection. Physicians in Savannah used this serum when they were called to see stricken individuals in sufficient time to allow its administration.

Frost did not write a separate account of his Savannah experience, but in January 1912 he published a general review of the subject of epidemic meningitis.[53] He carefully described the bacteriology, the epidemiology, the pathogenesis, the treatment, and the public health management of this disease. In his report he detailed the experience during this outbreak with antiserum therapy. Half of twenty-two afflicted persons treated with serum recovered, and results were most favorable when the agent was given within the first three days of the illness.

In the spring of 1912 a number of physicians in Baltimore, Maryland, noted a large number of cases of acute, febrile sore throat, the entity familiar to every parent as "strep throat." Between one and three thousand persons had become ill, and thirty or more had died as a result of complications of their infections. In conferring with one another, the Baltimore physicians had recognized that many of their patients drank milk from a single dairy. Today, we do not think of streptococcal sore throat as being spread by milk, but prior to universal pasteurization outbreaks due to contaminated milk were not uncommon. Indeed, the streptococcal organism can produce an infection of the udder of cows. By the time Frost was dispatched by the Public Health Service to investigate this outbreak, the dairy operator had been informed of the problem, had called in a sanitation expert, and had revised his pasteurization procedures. With this, the epidemic had ended rather promptly.

That the problem was now past did not deter Frost from making a careful study of the epidemic.[54] As he had done with typhoid and polio outbreaks, he carefully plotted the course of the epidemic, graphing the number of cases for ten days and showing that a sharp peak for customers of the dairy was followed two to three weeks later by a peak in the contacts of the initial cases. In families obtaining their milk from the source dairy, multiple cases were the rule; in families using milk from other dairies, single cases were commonest. Frost then inspected the dairy and its employees. He noted that the pasteurization equipment had not functioned properly prior to the epidemic and had, in fact, been out of service completely for five to seven days in order to accomplish repairs. Frost

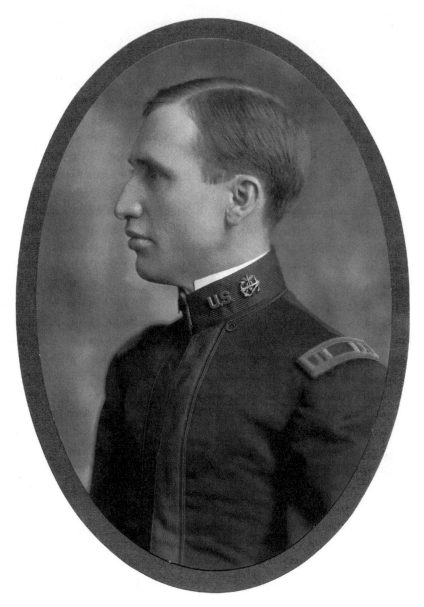

Figure 5.1. Wade Hampton Frost in his U.S. Public Health Service uniform. While undated, this studio photograph was undoubtedly taken during his assignment to the Hygienic Laboratory in Washington, D.C. Photograph is from the Claude Moore Health Sciences Library, University of Virginia Health Sciences Center, Charlottesville, VA: Wade Hampton Frost Archives, Box 6, Folder 27. Reproduced with permission, courtesy of the Historical Collection and Services of the Claude Moore Health Sciences Library.

concluded that the infecting bacteria were introduced into the milk before it reached the dairy, probably from a cow or cows with infected udders, and not removed because of breaks in the pasteurization procedure.

Frost became recognized by his public health colleagues and superiors as a competent and talented field investigator. Reflecting on this in 1975, Ernest Stebbins commented, "He was by that time one of the—if not the—outstanding epidemiologist of the Public Health Service."[55] With recognition came additional challenges. Frost was given other assignments unrelated to his major interests but presenting, nonetheless, public health problems needing attention. As noted, he investigated outbreaks of meningitis and septic sore throat. He wrote review papers on meningitis and plague, setting out appropriate control measures and, for the latter, the current status of immunization.[56] Frost's assignments not only provided him with laboratory and field experience. They stimulated him and led him to become knowledgeable in most of the major public health problems of the day. The breadth of knowledge he acquired during these few years was enormous.

Frost spent four and one-half years at the Hygienic Laboratory. Figure 5.1 shows him in his Public Health Service uniform at this time. His scientific output during those years was prodigious. He published twenty-two scientific papers totaling more than one thousand printed pages, complete with detailed tables and charts. During his Hygienic Laboratory years, Frost became a scientist and an epidemiologist; his keen mind amalgamated and integrated the analytic aspects of laboratory analysis with the field data collection aspects of shoe-leather epidemiology. Frost was being cast into the mold of a scientific epidemiologist, a mold still being shaped at the time, and into which he would later cast many students.

Frost worked hard during those Washington-based years, but he also enjoyed life in the nation's capital. While assigned there, he met Susan Noland Haxall, who would become his wife. The couple's courtship flourished, and marriage would not be far off.

6

Susan

Many medical men . . . admit the influence of
water [as a source of disease] without admitting
the special effect of the new element[s]
introduced into it.

—Wade Hampton Frost[1]

No documents survive to indicate just when and how Frost met
his bride-to-be, but some of the events can be surmised. Susan
Noland Haxall had left her home in Middleburg, Virginia, at
about age twenty-two and was living in an apartment in
Washington. Middleburg is located in Fauquier County about
fifteen miles northeast of Marshall—not far today, but a long
enough buggy ride at the end of the nineteenth century, so that
Frost and Susan Haxall had not met. The Haxall family home,
named Exning for the English town in which the Haxalls had
their genealogical roots, was located on the main road through
Middleburg (now US Route 50, the John Mosby Highway) to
the east of the town. Set back from the road at the end of a
tree-shaded drive and graced with a large veranda, it stands
today largely unchanged from the time that the Haxall's owned
it. Figure 6.1 shows Exning as it is today.

Susan Haxall operated a dancing school in Washington,
known as "Miss Haxall's Dancing Classes," teaching not only
ballroom dancing but also appropriate manners and etiquette
to young members of socially prominent families in the
nations's capital. She was a competent business woman, and
supported herself for seventeen years in this manner. She had
many relatives in Washington, and with them and their friends
had an active social life.

Frost enjoyed dancing, which he had learned while a student at Danville Military Institute, but he did not meet Susan in

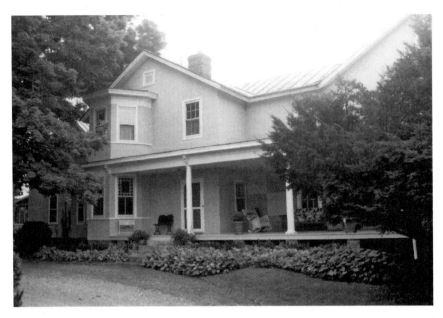

Figure 6.1. Exning, the Haxall family home in Middleburg, as it appeared in 2001. No alterations visible in this photograph have been made since it was occupied by the Haxalls. Photograph by the author.

that context, since her school was for children. They may, of course, have had enjoyable moments on the dance floor at one or another social function. They shared some common acquaintances, and most certainly met through one of them. Dr. Bolling M. Barton was a distant relative of the Haxalls. A widower, he lived with Susan's family at Exning for many of Susan's childhood years and was very close to the Haxall family. He was commonly called "Uncle" by Susan and her siblings, and upon his death was buried in a Haxall plot in the Sharon Cemetery in Middleburg. He in turn was a good friend of William T. Sedgwick. Barton introduced Sedgwick to the Haxall family at Exning, and he too became a family friend. Sedgwick was a sanitary engineer and a professor of biology and public health in a program that he founded at the Massachusetts Institute of Technology. He was one of the earliest and most prominent of American sanitarians. Although not a physician, he had a special interest in waterborne diseases.

During the winter of 1890–91, an epidemic of typhoid fever occurred in Lowell, Massachusetts. Sedgwick investigated it in what was probably the first application in North America of the techniques of the newly emergent science of bacteriology to the study of such a problem.[2]

Sedgwick was a member of the advisory board of the Hygienic Laboratory. His interests and expertise brought him into contact with Frost at a time when much of the latter's laboratory studies were focused on the potability of water drawn from the Potomac River. Thus, the two men shared a common professional interest; they also became friends and shared common friends, including Barton and others. Although the time and place of Frost and Susan Haxall's meeting are not known, it was clear to their daughter, Susan Frost Parrish, that her parents met through the Barton-Sedgwick connection.[3] There were additional family ties that were probably important in fostering the relationship of the couple. Hugh Cumming was then a Public Health Service surgeon stationed in Washington at the Hygienic Laboratory where he worked alongside Frost in the same laboratory division. A University of Virginia graduate, he was a distant "cousin" of Susan Haxall. Later he would become one of the couple's close friends as well as Frost's superior officer as Surgeon General. One must suppose that Cumming might also have played a role in bringing the couple together.

Susan Noland Haxall came from a distinguished family with its roots in England and colonial Virginia. Her genealogy can be traced back five generations to John Haxall, who was born in 1661 and died in 1751. He lived in Exning in Suffolk, England. His second son William married Catherine Newton, also of Exning. They had fourteen children. Their youngest son, Philip, who was born in 1770, emigrated to Virginia, settling in Petersburg in 1786. There, with two of his brothers, William and Henry, he founded the Petersburg Mills. In June, 1809, he and his brother, William, purchased the Columbian Mills in Richmond and renamed it Haxall Mills. Philip married Clara Walker of Richmond. Their eighth child and fifth son, Bolling

Walker Haxall, was born in 1814. He married Ann Triplett, and they had three sons, Richard Barton Haxall, William Henry Haxall, and Bolling Walker Haxall, Junior. These three brothers took over the operation of Haxall Mills from their father. The business prospered and the Haxall brothers became men of wealth and social prominence. The mill, which shipped flour world-wide, burned down following the fall of Richmond during the Civil War, but the Haxall family weathered the loss and rebuilt it. The senior Bolling Haxall died in 1885.

Bolling Walker Haxall Jr., who was born in 1851, was educated at a gymnasium in Germany and at the Sorbonne in Paris, France. He moved to Middleburg, Virginia, after the Civil War and married Lavenia Anderson Noland, also known as Lena, two years his junior, on August 10, 1874. She was the daughter of Burr Powell Noland, who had served as a major in the Confederate army and was practicing law in Middleburg. The Noland family was one of Middleburg's most prominent. Bolling and Lavenia Haxall built a comfortable and gracious home east of Middleburg on what is now known as the John Mosby Highway, which they named Exning. They had three daughters and a son. Susan Noland Haxall was their eldest. Her siblings were Ann Triplett, Bolling Walker, who was killed in World War I, and Louise Triplett Harris, known as Ouida.[4] Exning, the home they built, would serve as the Haxall homestead for the next three generations.

What sort of person was this woman whom Frost would ask to be his wife? Four years older than her suitor, she was an attractive young woman, well-educated, feminine, and polished in her social graces. Figure 6.2 is a studio portrait photograph of her at about this time. Susan loved antiques and gardening—proper interests for a young woman of those times. Talkative by nature, she was an adept conversationalist, charming all she met. She had a gift for setting people at ease. She was, in the words of her daughter, "a social animal." Moreover, she was a clever raconteuse with a flair for wit and humor. "She could really roll them in the aisles. If you don't have a sense of humor, you lack one of the most essential ingredients [of graciousness]."[5] At the same time, she could be

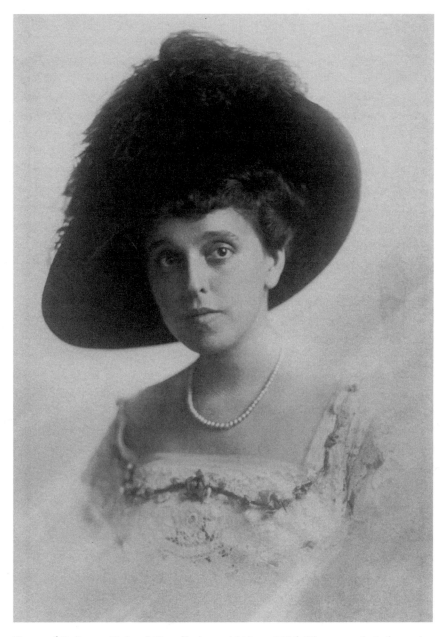

Figure 6.2. Susan Noland Haxall about 1913 or 1914. Photograph is from the Claude Moore Health Sciences Library, University of Virginia Health Sciences Center, Charlottesville, VA: Wade Hampton Frost Archives, Box 6, Folder 24. Reproduced with permission, courtesy of the Historical Collection and Services of the Claude Moore Health Sciences Library.

strong willed. Her daughter, reminiscing, remembered Susan Frost as gentle but having a quick temper.[6]

Susan Haxall was also a woman of courage with a strong sense of justice and moral obligation. In about 1910 a white man was murdered in Middleburg. A crippled, African-American man was convicted of the crime and sentenced to be executed. Tension in the community was high; the African-American population was sure of his innocence, and Susan found their arguments convincing. She traveled to Richmond, the state capital, and obtained a pardon of the convicted man from the governor. Later the actual killer was apprehended and convicted. The members of the local African-American Baptist church gave Susan a mahogany table to express their gratitude.[7]

Frost was soon enamored. She also found him attractive, and their relationship flourished. Susan liked to sew, and she made portieres to curtain off a portion of Frost's apartment.[8] Later, when they established a home in Baltimore, she made all of the curtains and slipcovers for the furniture.

As much in love and compatible as the two of them were, they had not been spawned in the same pond. The Haxall family members were conscious of their deep roots in what one might call the "upper social class" of colonial Virginia. The Haxalls cared a great deal about their background, and it was of particular interest to Susan. However, when the words "upper class" were used in questioning the Frost's daughter, Susan Frost Parrish, she bristled:

> May I object. . . . I would say [they were] people who are well-bred, perhaps, . . . or who came from "old families." It isn't that [the] term is incorrect, but I think that they would object to it. Yes, I think that is true.[9]

The Frost family, on the other hand, was poor, but its members are remembered as intelligent and well-educated.[10] Their roots in South Carolina were also deep and aristocratic, but they had been torn from the southern earth by the Civil War and the reconstruction period that followed it. Wade Hampton Frost was comfortable in both worlds; his University of Virginia education had prepared him well for life in Washington and life with Susan Noland Haxall. In fact, as time passed and with the deaths of his parents, Frost became more and more a member of the Haxall clan, closer to many of its members than to some of his own brothers and sisters.

The Frost-Haxall romance flourished, but it was not to progress without impediments. Public Health Service officers were and still are, like military officers, subject to reassignment to meet the needs of the service. Wade Hampton Frost was transferred from Washington, with its proximity to Susan Haxall, to Cincinnati, Ohio, a full day's train travel distant in that era before commercial aviation.

"I must go across the river, over the hills where the trail leads west," sang Johnny Appleseed, the folk hero romanticized as having brought apples to Ohio. As colonists surged westward beyond the Appalachian Mountains, the Ohio River became one of the most important routes leading west to the new frontier. In 1778 George Rogers Clark led a military campaign that assured control of the river by the new American nation. Ten years later Lasantiville was founded on the north bank of the river; it was renamed Cincinnati in 1790. The Queen City, as it was christened by Henry Wadsworth Longfellow, rapidly became a major port, increased in its importance in the early nineteenth century when canals were built to link the Ohio River with Lake Erie.

Years and decades passed. The land of opportunity lay in the west. In the mid nineteenth century the California gold rush increased the stream of pioneers. Cincinnati and other midwestern cities grew. North America's rivers assumed even greater importance, and many cities flourished on their banks. And so also did the diseases they often harbored.

In November 1891 Guy Ward Mallon married Hannah Neil, the daughter of a prominent Columbus, Ohio, businessman. A recent graduate of Yale University, he had followed his Eli years by studying law in Cincinnati, where his father was a respected lawyer, judge, and colleague of Alonso Taft. The first of the couple's nine children was born in August 1892, a son, named Guy Ward Mallon Jr., after his father. Six months later, on February 20, 1893, the infant boy died of cholera.[11] The Ohio River brought not only prosperity to Cincinnati and the Mallon family; it brought waterborne disease and the death of an infant son.

The United States was just beginning to keep national health records in the early twentieth century, but even without such documentation it was evident that waterborne diseases fostered by pollution of stream and river with sewage were a major problem in the Midwest. Typhoid fever death rates and epidemics, such as that investigated by Frost in Williamson, were bellwethers, for typhoid was well known to most doctors and could be identified with reasonable accuracy by blood tests. The introduction of filtration plants, providing some degree of water purification for many cities along the Ohio River, including Pittsburgh, Cincinnati, and Louisville, resulted in a decrease in the typhoid death rate in those cities from 90.5 per 100,000 in 1906 to 15.3 per 100,000 in 1914.[12]

In 1910 the United States Public Health Service inaugurated a study of interstate waterway pollution under the direction of Allan J. McLaughlin. Two years later the American effort was joined by Canada with the establishment of a joint commission, headed by McLaughlin. Congress acted in August 1912, extending the purview of the Public Health Service to include "sanitation and sewage and the pollution . . . of the navigable streams and lakes of the United States." In 1913 funds were appropriated for the establishment of a field station for the study of water pollution. With this, a new laboratory and field station were opened in Cincinnati using the facilities of a marine hospital that was no longer in service. Wade Hampton Frost was chosen as the director of the new unit.[13]

Mortality statistics were collected in the United States by the Bureau of the Census beginning at the dawn of the twentieth century, with an increasing number of reporting sites added each year. In 1913, the year in which the Cincinnati station opened, the overall mortality for those areas reporting to the national registry was 1,407.4 per 100,000. For typhoid fever, the death rate was 17.9 per 100,000. For diarrheal disease in infants less than two years of age, it was 75.2 per 100,000. In the same year, Hamilton County, Ohio, which largely comprises Cincinnati, the overall death rate was 1,171.3 per 100,000. For typhoid and infant diarrhea the rates were 16.8 per 100,000 and 55.4 per 100,000.[14] Cincinnati's problems with waterborne illnesses were reasonably representative of those of the country as a whole. Studies in that river city would benefit all Americans. That Cincinnati had fewer typhoid and diarrheal illnesses than other localities was attributed by Frost to the fact that Cincinnati filtered its drinking water.[15]

Frost summarized the purposes of the Ohio River project and the approaches that were to be used.

> Briefly stated the object of the current investigation of the Ohio River is to determine the amount and character of the domestic sewage and other wastes discharged into the river, their immediate and remote effects upon the stream, the natural processes of stream-purification, and, as the most important and ultimate object, to study the relations between pollution of the river and the health of those resident upon its banks. Such a broad problem must necessarily be approached from many different angles, and the investigation as being conducted includes the following principal subdivisions: Studies of the physical characteristics and habitation of the watershed; careful studies of the volume and velocity of the river; detailed estimates of the amounts and kinds of wastes which it receives; extended bacteriological and chemical analyses of the river water at critical points; studies of the plankton life; and analyses of the vital statistics of Ohio River communities, with special reference to such effects as may be ascribed to the pollution of the river. In a general way the effects produced both upon rivers and upon the public health by sewage-pollution are already known, and it is not expected that the present investigation will develop any facts of new or startling import. Its aim is rather to follow the lines of definite effects, determining them so far as possible in a quantitative way, hoping in this way to establish some broad principles which may be generally applicable.[16]

In 1815, David Kilgour, a prosperous merchant, had built a stately mansion overlooking the Ohio River on one of Cincinnati's many hills. In 1882 the Kilgour home was purchased by the government for use as a marine hospital. The house provided space for administrative offices, and additional buildings were erected on the property for patient wards.

While initially accommodating as many as five hundred patients, the occupancy of the hospital rapidly declined, and when it had closed in 1905 it had only eight patients. Thus, it was available and provided generous space for the new field station.

Frost arrived in Cincinnati in the summer of 1913. He was knowledgeable about stream pollution—it had been a major focus of his work at the National Hygienic Laboratory— and was well prepared to take on the challenges of this new assignment. Four other Public Health Service officers were assigned to work with him. Paul Preble, Lewis R. Thompson, Joseph Bolton, and H. F. Smith were medical officers of the Public Health Service assigned to Cincinnati. Additional sanitary experts were added to the team. They included sanitary engineers John K. Hoskins, Ralph E. Tarbett, and Harold W. Streeter; pharmacist F. A. Southard; plankton expert William C. Purdy; bacteriologists E. M. Meyer, H. M. Campbell, Milton V. Veldee, and E. E. Smith; and chemists J. A. Carven and Emery J. Theriault. Assistance to the group was provided by C. E. Ellsworth, District Engineer of the United States Geological Survey, and by Earl B. Phelps, a chemist and bacteriologist who had been a professor at the Massachusetts Institute of Technology with Sedgwick and a hydrographer with the Geological Survey before joining the Public Health Service in 1913. Frost established five branch laboratories along the river to collect and initially process water samples. He arranged for the remodeling of the Marine Hospital facilities into appropriate laboratory space. He found living quarters for himself about one and one-half miles from the station at 1322 East McMillan Avenue.

Frost brought more than knowledge of waterborne diseases and administrative and laboratory skills to the Cincinnati station he directed. In the worlds of his water quality colleague Abel Wolman:

> He was the intellectual mentor. His curiosity spilled over from the medical field . . . to great advantage in shedding [an] intellectual look on the problems in the environment. . . . There was no prior productivity in

that field except of a very general nature. . . . What came out of it under his stimulation was concreteness, specificity of high quality, quantitative evaluation, and the creation of principles that were [previously] lacking, because this was his kind of a mind. He was always on a search, not for another little paper, . . . but [for] an underlying principle.[17]

Frost's concern with both quantitative analyses and the principles underlying the spread of waterborne disease are well illustrated by a paper he published in the *Journal of the American Water Works Association* in 1915.[18] While not blazing new paths of public health thought, this paper nicely reflects Frost's thinking. He noted that drinking water, whether taken from surface or subsurface sources, had been in contact with soil and therefore potentially in contact with sewage. Taking typhoid as his example, he noted that it is caused by a bacillus shed in human feces and urine and that there are no animal reservoirs. Culture of this organism from water is difficult, but coliform bacilli are readily isolated from water and can be taken as an index of either human or animal fecal contamination. The presence of coliform bacilli shows

only the extent of pollution with intestinal discharges in general; they do not distinguish between pollution with intestinal discharges from lower animals which are not subject to infection with typhoid bacilli, and the much more dangerous pollution from human sources. They still further fail to distinguish between human discharges actually containing typhoid bacilli and discharges free from this specific infection.[19]

While embracing the principle of using coliform bacilli as a surrogate index of pollution with sewage, Frost clearly expressed his reservations concerning its quantification and application.

More than a decade later, Frost reflected on the state of knowledge in the area of water purification.[20] He noted three needs: (1) objective measurable criteria for water purity, (2) precise knowledge of the reliability and efficiency of water purification processes, and (3) the quantitative role of upstream pollution by settlements discharging raw sewage into the water. Here again, Frost's concern with the application of quantification to established principles is evident.

The blossoming romance between Frost and Susan Haxall had been interrupted, but not derailed, when Frost was assigned to head the field station studying water pollution in Cincinnati. The couple corresponded by mail, and Frost visited Susan in Washington when he could. In the fall of 1914, he asked her to marry him, and by Christmas she was telling friends and family the good news. Their friend William Sedgwick wrote to Susan upon hearing of their engagement:

> Few things in life have given me keener pleasure than the great good news which [your] letter to my wife brought to me today. I have believed for a good while that Dr. Frost was deeply attached to you, for in the . . . references he made to you I seemed to detect a regard so strong that it could have but one meaning. And then when I saw you like a beautiful siren in your lovely apartment in the Farragut I couldn't help feeling that your heart too had a rare chamber in it reserved for the right possessor.[21]

The following day, Sedgwick wrote to Frost in Cincinnati:

> I had suspected your devotion to Susan Haxall (for who could resist her winning and thoroughly feminine personality) and I had also suspected that she must be difficult to win. . . . It's a wonderful, and in many ways a fearsome thing, this affection and this lifelong attachment of a man and a maid and you are both old enough to realize that.[22]

Life itself is often less straightforward than one's plans for life. And so it was for the engaged couple. Susan developed acute appendicitis shortly before their engagement, and her recovery was slow. Public announcement of their engagement was delayed until after the new year. In January, Henry Frost wrote to his son:

> I see the announcement of your engagement in the Sun today. . . . I have felt very sorry for you, knowing that you must have been disappointed at the delay in your plans, but I hope now for a speedy consummation.[23]

Sedgwick advised them to "decide on an early marriage, without the wearing details of a formal & public 'wedding.'"[24] "Carry her off almost by force to a new environment," he wrote, a suggestion supported also by Susan's friend and distant relative Bolling Barton. With Susan wanting more and more time to attend to what she considered important arrangements and Frost pushing for an early wedding, the couple finally were married on February 15, 1915, in a private ceremony at Exning, the Haxall home in Middleburg, Virginia. Susan's two sisters and her brother, with their spouses, were among the thirteen guests, as were a few other Haxall relatives. The Frost family was represented by Frost's sisters; his parents may have been too ill to attend at that time. All of the guests signed the prayer book that Susan held in her hands during the ceremony.[25] Frost was then two weeks shy of his thirty-fifth birthday; Susan was five days shy of her thirty-ninth.

Susan joined her husband in Cincinnati, where the couple found an apartment in a building named "The Maplewood," on Bryant Avenue in the Clifton neighborhood of that city. Their life in Cincinnati was a happy one. Correspondence between Frost and his father, of which the letters from the latter survive, kept Frost apprized of events in Marshall and of the dwindling health of his parents.[26] Susan remained in touch with her parents, and the couple made occasional visits to their Fauquier County, Virginia, families. In the late fall of 1915, Susan was delighted to find she was pregnant. Her pregnancy was uneventful, and as her time drew near she returned to her family home, Exning, where her daughter, Susan Haxall Frost, was born on June 11, 1916.

Susan Frost returned to Cincinnati to rejoin her husband, bringing her infant daughter with her. Eva Anderson, who had worked for the senior Frost family in Marshall for three years, went to Cincinnati to help care for the new baby. She remained with Wade Hampton and Susan Frost from then on and become a regular fixture in the Frost household.

When her baby was about six weeks old, Susan took her first outing, her release from the long confinement customary for new mothers at that time. She went for an automobile ride with a Mrs. Morrison, a Cincinnati friend. An accident occurred. Susan was thrown from the car, which then rolled over and pinned her beneath it. She suffered several fractured vertebrae. In fact, from that time on she had a deformity of her back, had frequent back pain, and wore a series of back braces.[27]

Frost's studies of the water quality of the Ohio River were not always welcomed. He established laboratory stations along the Ohio River and charged them with sampling municipally supplied drinking water and assessing the suitability of the sanitary activities of towns along the river. A quantitative scoring system was set up, with a perfect score of 100 being possible. Up to forty points could be awarded for the potability of municipal drinking water; up to twenty-five for sewage treatment; the remaining thirty-five for other aspects of the municipality's sanitary systems. This scoring system was augmented by surveys of the prevalence of typhoid fever in riverside communities.[28]

As water filtration systems were installed in the Ohio Valley, a low-cost system known as the "Smith System of Natural Filtration" was aggressively promoted by its vendors to riverside communities. This system relied on a perforated grid placed on the river bottom and covered with sand to filter the water. Although data had accumulated to demonstrate the unreliability of this system, its low cost continued to make it attractive. The city of Wheeling, West Virginia, had been trying for several years to find the funds necessary to build an efficient water filtration system. The choice of system was then put to a popular vote, and when the ballots were tallied, the citizens had chosen the low-cost Smith system. Wheeling's City Engineer, C. B. Cook, was disturbed by this action, and on November 11, 1914, he wrote to Frost asking for data from the nearby town of Parkersburg, West Virginia, which had been using the Smith filtration system for two years. Frost wrote a detailed reply, sent through the office of the Public Health Service Surgeon General, in which he provided in great detail the data collected in Parkersburg as part of the survey of Ohio River community sanitary activities. He provided bacteriologic data for Wheeling's as yet untreated water, for Cincinnati's water then being purified with a modern filtration system, and for Parkersburg's water filtered using the Smith system. The data clearly demonstrated that the Smith system, while removing some bacteria, failed to live up to the standards that were achieved in Cincinnati. He concluded his letter by saying:

> These figures speak for themselves and give an idea of the Parkersburg supply more significant and valuable than an expression of personal opinion. . . . [However,] in my opinion the results fully justify classing the Parkersburg supply as unsafe. . . . I do not see how any [other] conclusion can be drawn.[29]

The citizens of Parkersburg learned of this letter, and they were not happy. John Marshall, a Parkersburg attorney, fired off an angry letter to Rupert Blue, Surgeon General of the Public Health Service, on behalf of the Board of Commerce of that community. After a review of the data, Blue replied that

> The data contained in the letter of Dr. Frost [and] the facts stated therein are not only reliable as regards their accuracy, but are sufficient to form the basis of the opinion rendered in respect to the quality of the Parkersburg water supply.[30]

Frost not only carried his campaign for understanding the need for water purification to the citizenry of Wheeling and Parkersburg. He spoke to the region's health professionals. He addressed the subject at the Mississippi Valley Medical Association meeting in Cincinnati in October 1914, and again at a meeting of the Ohio Medical Association in Cleveland, Ohio, in May 1916.[31] He opened the latter presentation by pointing out that, "in every inhabited country the surface waters almost invariably become more or less polluted with human excreta," and then discussed in detail the measures that could be taken to protect the health of the community in this situation.

In the summer of 1916, polio struck New York City with unprecedented ferocity. More than nine thousand cases of paralytic disease occurred. The annual case rate climbed to 28.5 per 100,000, 3.5 times the highest case rate previously observed in the United States. Near panic ensued.[32]

As noted in chapter 5, poliomyelitis is an ancient disease—it is represented in antiquity on an Egyptian stela carved about 3,500 years ago.[33] Infantile paralysis it was called, for it was most commonly seen as a rare, severe, paralytic disease of infants. Then, at the end of the nineteenth century, outbreaks began to occur among adults, with a major epidemic in Stockholm, Sweden, in 1887.

Frost was an expert on polio. He had worked on polio during his time at the Hygienic Laboratory, where he had confirmed its viral causation. In the field, he had participated in the investigation of epidemics in Iowa, Cincinnati, and in New York State. He had served as chairman of the American Medical Association Committee on Methods for the Control of Poliomyelitis and led the analysis of national data on polio incidence. In fact, Frost had made major contributions to our understanding of the natural history of polio. It was he who had understood more clearly than any of his predecessor that polio was a frequent childhood infection, usually mild and unnoticed, rarely accompanied by paralysis. Only the occasional iceberg-tip severe case was noticed. Those children who had mild infections acquired immunity, however, and remained protected from polio for the remainder of their lives. But during these mild infections, they passed poliovirus in their stools. With poor sanitation the virus found its way into water systems— just as typhoid bacilli did in Williamson, West Virginia. With better sanitation, virus did not spread, so individuals reached adulthood without immunity. Then, when a break in sanitation occurred, outbreaks of disease followed. Now, adults were meeting the virus for the first time, and most adults infected with poliovirus develop major disease, frequently paralytic.

New York City's health commissioner at the time of the 1916 polio outbreak was Haven Emerson, an early pioneer in the field of public health. The control efforts mounted by the city's health department were monumental. They included placarding and quarantining all dwellings in which a case occurred and placing a travel ban on all children sixteen years-old or younger unless they were certified as living in a home free of the disease. Hermann Biggs, now having moved from New York City to become health Commissioner for the State of New York, had established quarantine and isolation as firm elements of public health control in that city while he served as its chief medical officer. In few other locations was this strategy pursued with such zeal.[34] The rationale for applying this approach to polio is hard to understand, for Frost and others had already provided convincing evidence that clinically recognizable cases represented only a fraction of the actual cases in an epidemic. Moreover, clinically evident cases were rare among close family contacts of patients. Quarantine measures could contribute little to the control of spread of infection in this situation.

The Public Health Service offered assistance to New York. The mayor of New York City was quick to accept. Two teams were dispatched by the Public Health Service, one headed by Charles E. Banks charged with working with Emerson to enforce quarantine and travel regulations in the city. The second, charged with conducting a scientific investigation of the epidemic, was headed by Claude H. Lavinder.[35] Eight years Frost's senior, Lavinder was also a Virginian. Like Frost he had attended Randolph-Macon college and then the University of Virginia, where he had earned his medical degree before entering the Public Health Service. Lavinder knew Frost, and it was not long before he had summoned his younger, expert colleague to the investigative team.[36] In addition to Frost, Lavinder's team included Edward Francis, James P. Leake, William Draper, and Allen W. Freeman. Others joined for short periods of duty with the project. Of those assigned, only Frost had prior experience and expertise with polio. Freeman was one of Frost's Cincinnati colleagues.

In response to the call of duty, Frost went to New York. Susan and their young daughter returned to the Haxall family home in Middleburg, Virginia, taking a nurse with them from Cincinnati to assist in caring for the young mother who was still convalescent from her back injury. In a letter dated October 2, 1916, Frost's father reported that he had heard from Susan's mother that Susan and the baby had made the journey without difficulty and were comfortably settled at Exning and doing well.[37] They would not return to Cincinnati.

New York was then the second largest city in the world with a population of 5.6 million—no small challenge for an epidemiologic investigation. Between 1909 and 1915, the United States death rate from poliomyelitis had varied between 1.0 and 2.7 per 100,000, corresponding to about 2,000 deaths nationwide. Case reports were incomplete; the best estimates put the annual figures at between 5,000 and 12,000 for each year nationally. In New York City, the annual case rate had varied between 5.8 and 14.4 per 100,000; during the 1916 epidemic, the case rate reached 185 per 100,000. There were approximately 9,000 cases of polio in New York City during that outbreak. If one includes the surrounding areas, the total reached an estimated 23,000 cases. The epidemic appeared to have started in Brooklyn, spreading first to lower Manhattan where it reached its greatest intensity, and then to Staten Island and areas surrounding the city.[38]

Lavinder, Frost, and their colleagues went to work. An office was established in the New York City Health Department. Polio had been made a reportable disease in 1909, and daily reports of new cases were available to the team. Freeman and Frost took primary responsibility for the statistical data. Others of the team investigated individual cases to confirm diagnoses and to collect specimens for laboratory analysis. A detailed study was carried out in Staten Island.

At the end of the summer, the epidemic waned, as have all polio epidemics before and since. Frost returned to his duties in Cincinnati. Susan remained at Exning with their daughter, and Frost moved to smaller living quarters. Yet there was more to be done with the polio epidemic. Mountains of data had been collected, and a final report was needed, even though the team had dispersed. But war was brewing, and it was difficult for those working on the report to come together for the work. They had no more than two brief opportunities for conferences related to the task. In the end, Freeman and Frost assembled most of the statistical information and wrote related sections in Cincinnati. Lavinder, at the National Hygienic Laboratory in Washington, wrote the final document, largely by assembling separate sections written by the three men.[39]

Despite the difficulties, the final document is monumental in scope and insightful in its conclusions. It stands as a classic in its field.

Reflecting on his experience with polio culminating with the New York City investigations, Frost made a substantially definitive statement concerning the transmission of poliomyelitis. First noting that only monkeys and rabbits among animals could be infected and that they could not be considered likely vectors, he commented that early work had shown that transmission by insects was possible only "under highly artificial conditions." He concluded (emphasizing his words with italics):

> *On the whole, the experimental evidence . . . points to the conclusion that poliomyelitis is a contagious disease, spread from person to person through interchange of infectious secretions, the sources of infection being the clinically definite and clinically indefinite acute cases of poliomyelitis, convalescents, and passive human carriers.*[40]

It is modern understanding of that concept so elegantly articulated by Frost that has permitted the surveillance needed to certify eradication of polio from much of the world following vaccination campaigns.

Frost resumed his post in Cincinnati. His work there continued for another year and one-half before it was interrupted by the exigencies of war. Even after Frost's career had turned down other roads to meet other challenges, he remained interested in water quality. He remained nominally in charge of the Cincinnati station after he moved to Baltimore, and he continued as a consultant to the station and the Public Health Service after he had resigned his commission. In 1926 he published a summary review of the Public Health Service's activity in the area of water quality.[41] In 1925, 1926, and 1927 he attended the annual conferences of the state and territorial health officers of the Public Health Service and participated in symposia discussing water pollution.[42] His studies of water pollution were, for Frost, important not only for their potential impact on public health, but also for his personal development in the arena of data analysis. To quote his colleague, Kenneth Maxcy, "As director it was Frost's responsibility to organize and correlate these studies."[43] With his assignment in Cincinnati, Frost stepped boldly onto an analytic path that he would follow throughout the rest of his career and life.

7

Dread Diseases

As compared with the clinical manifestations of a disease, its epidemiological characteristics, which can be put together only in a conceptual way, are more difficult to comprehend but not less distinctive.

—Wade Hampton Frost[1]

Charles Dickens characterized tuberculosis as a "dread disease, in which the struggle between soul and body is so gradual, quiet, and solemn, and the results so sure, that day by day and grain by grain, the mortal part wastes and withers away, so that the spirit grows light and sanguine."[2] Wade Hampton Frost met tuberculosis in November 1917, and that encounter surely had an impact on his spirit if not his mortal part.

In 1914 Europe became engulfed in the maelstrom of World War I. When a German submarine sank the Lusitania on May 7, 1915, with the loss of more than one thousand lives, including 128 Americans, anti-German sentiment began to mount in North America. Continuing tension was fired by increasingly frequent attacks on Atlantic shipping, and the United States entered the fray by declaring war on Germany on April 6, 1917. War meant mobilization, and the Public Health Service was included in this rush to war.

On April 3, 1917, President Woodrow Wilson issued an executive order incorporating the Public Health Service into the military forces of the United States. The pollution of the Ohio River seemed unimportant in that moment, and work at the Cincinnati field station came to a halt. Of much greater urgency were the many public-health-related issues raised by mobilizing and training a large army in hastily constructed camps. Public Health Service Surgeon General Rupert Blue was ready to assign his officers to this duty, but there were no funds available to support this activity. The American Red Cross stepped into the breach and offered funds to establish a Bureau of Sanitary Services within its organization to accomplish the needed work. Blue assigned Frost, who had ably demonstrated his administrative skills in Cincinnati, to organize and direct this office. Frost promptly reported to Washington and plunged into the task.[3] On April 21, 1917, he was promoted to the rank of surgeon.

The International Committee of the Red Cross, known to all simply as the Red Cross, was founded in Switzerland in 1864. Its founders were concerned about the lack of care for prisoners and other victims of war, and the original purpose of the Red Cross was to provide medical care and assistance to prisoners of war and refugees displaced by warring armies. Later this mission was expanded to include many types of disaster relief. The American National Red Cross was organized by Clara Barton in 1881 and chartered by the United States Congress in 1900 and again in 1905. In addition to providing medical care and aid to the victims of war, the American Red Cross was specifically charged with serving as a medium of communication between military personnel and their families and with providing domestic disaster relief. The bureau being organized by Frost at the Washington offices of the Red Cross would be primarily concerned with the domestic public health issues of mobilizing an army and sending it into the battlefield. As Frost saw it, wartime health issues were not limited to those of soldiers and sailors but also pertained to the war-disrupted civilian population. In his words:

> The conditions of war . . . impose additional burdens . . . as a result of the concentration of population in and around military encampments and industrial centers. Additional public health problems will arise in the civil population as the war progresses . . . and certainly after the war a great expansion of public health activities will be necessary for reconstruction.
>
> At the same time the forces of skilled sanitarians . . . have already been considerably reduced and will be still further and greatly reduced . . . by the withdrawal of trained sanitarians for service in the military forces.[4]

Frost was not destined to spend a long time at this Washington assignment, for in November 1917 he was found to have pulmonary tuberculosis. As had his brother before him, he went to Asheville, North Carolina, to rest and "cure."

Tuberculosis is an ancient disease, well documented in Egyptian and Andean mummies. Yet the world had moved forward, and humans had conquered many of the infections that plagued their early history. How could Frost have contracted tuberculosis in the twentieth century? In fact, this ancient plague has often been a common disease, sometimes engulfing entire continents. It reached epidemic proportions in Europe and North America during the eighteenth and nineteenth centuries.[5] Death rates in cities reached 800 to 1,000 per 100,000 population each year at the end of the nineteenth century.[6] It is reasonable to assume that new cases were occurring at an incidence rate of about twice those figures, 1,600 to 2,000 per 100,000 a year. By the time of Frost's diagnosis, the mortality rate in the United States had fallen to about 130 per 100,000. For comparison, the new case rate in the United States was 5.1 per 100,000 in 2003; the death rate for 2001 was 0.3 per 100,000.[7] In Frost's day, tuberculosis was no longer the "Captain of Death," as John Bunyon had named it in 1660, but it remained a disease of considerable consequence. It was not uncommon, and the mortality rate overall remained at about 15 percent, even with the best medical care available in that pre-antibiotic era. The Frost family was not unique in being visited by the "white plague."

Attempts to treat tuberculosis go back to antiquity. The first-century Roman physician, Pliny the Elder, recommended wolf's liver steeped in wine; alternatively he favored shavings from the hoof of an ox, ashes of the tongues of pigs or the lungs of deer, both in wine. John Keats was treated with horseback rides and blood letting. Sea voyages were a not uncommon prescription. In the nineteenth century special hospitals for the treatment of tuberculosis were first opened. Among them were specialized facilities that became known as sanatoria. In 1859 Herman Brehmer opened his Heilanstalt Sanatorium at Goerbersdorf in the Silesian Mountains of Prussia. Brehmer theorized that tuberculosis was caused by enlarged lungs, and he reasoned that living at high altitude with its reduced oxygen would shrink the lungs and heal tuberculous lesions. At his sanatorium he instituted a regimen of vigorous exercise and mountain climbing. Brehmer's pupil Peter Detwiler opened a similar sanatorium in Falkenstein, near Frankfort, Germany, in 1867. There he introduced rest to the treatment of this disease, while continuing what became known as "the outdoor life." Other sanatoria followed and certain locations became known as health promoting, including Davos, Switzerland, the setting for Thomas Mann's *Magic Mountain*. In North America, Joseph Gleitsman established the first American mountain sanatorium for the treatment of tuberculosis in Asheville, North Carolina, in 1875. This location in the Great Smokey Mountains soon became famous, and as the cold winds of November 1917 ushered in winter, Frost joined many others in repairing there for his "cure."[8]

There is no direct information concerning Frost's treatment in Asheville, but a number of logical deductions can be made that give us insights into his experience there. He placed himself under the care of Dr. Charles L. Minor, a leading tuberculosis specialist in Asheville at that time. Minor, like Frost, was a graduate of the University of Virginia, receiving his medical degree in 1888. He initially practiced in Washington, D.C., but in 1894 he contracted tuberculosis and moved to the salubrious environs of Asheville. After recovering his health, he stayed there and resumed his practice, limiting his work to the care of patients with tuberculosis. He enjoyed a national reputation in this field, published a number of scholarly articles on the subject, and was a founding member of the National Tuberculosis Association (now the American Lung Association) and the society's thirteenth president.[9]

Over the course of the first few decades of the twentieth century, sanatoria evolved into specialized tuberculosis hospitals, but in many popular "cure" locations they were places of residence rather than hospitals, with care being provided by local physicians who were usually specialists in treating tuberculosis. This appears to have been the normal mode for Minor's patients in Asheville. The proper care of patients with this disease was also under evolution, earlier mandates for vigorous exercise giving way to enforced bed rest, sometimes extreme in its totality. A letter to Frost from William T. Sedgwick, Frost's friend and public health and sanitation colleague and a professor at the Massachusetts Institute of Technology, reads:

> We are all thinking of you with envy! Just think, to be ordered to lie still and have the time of your life, or what would be such a time if only you had Susan and Susette with you. I look back upon the summer when I was ordered to keep still as one of the pleasantest of my life.[10]

Minor was a moderate in his use of exercise, and we can assume that Frost was subjected to a moderate regimen including hours spent reclining at rest in the sun and long if leisurely walks on mountain paths. On May 11, 1914, not long before he cared for Frost, Minor read a paper at the thirty-third annual meeting of the American Clinical and Climatological Association in Washington, D.C. His presentation was reported in the *Medical Record*, a leading professional journal of the day. He was quoted as saying, "Formerly tuberculosis patients were permitted to over-exercise; to-day there [is] a tendency to go to the other extreme." He then cited the need for hope and encouragement provided by relaxing rest prescriptions, provided guidelines for allowing walks of up to an hour depending on the patient's maximum afternoon temperature, and said, "As to fatigue, a little healthy tire [has] no significance, but to get really fatigued [is] bad."[11]

That activity was governed by small differences in afternoon temperatures was the rule in the care of consumptives at that time. Mann called the thermometer "the silent sister."[12] Minor's injunctions were reported as:

> Temperature was the best guide to detect over-exertion. If the temperature in the afternoon was as high as 99.4° F., the patient could be gotten up in the morning only, then if he progressed properly in the afternoon, and finally all day. With a temperature of 99.6° F., . . . it might often be wise to allow him up in a reclining chair for an hour or so in the morning.[13]

Details of Frost's illness are not available, but he could not have been very ill, for his stay in Asheville was short by the standards of that time. Maxcy, his colleague and friend, called Frost's disease "incipient," a term commonly used to describe early tuberculosis at the time he wrote (1941) but lacking in precise definition.[14] In fact, there is substantial reason to believe that this episode was not his first encounter with the "dread disease." As noted in chapter 4, Phillip E. Sartwell, a professor of epidemiology at Johns Hopkins School of Hygiene and Public Health, speculated that Frost had had tuberculosis "some time during his educational career or before."[15] One must wonder if the year between studies at Randolph Macon and the University of Virginia was spent at home because of this illness. The post-pubertal, late-teen years constitute a time of life when child-hood infections with the tubercle bacillus are likely to erupt into active disease, a fact demonstrated in a landmark study to which Frost would serve as a major consultant in his later years.[16]

Frost spent only a relatively brief six months at Asheville before returning for reassignment. The usual course of treatment in American centers was not different from that pre-scribed by Dr. Hofrat for Frost's fictional contemporary, Hans Castorp, in Thomas Mann's *The Magic Mountain*. "But I tell you straight away, a case like yours doesn't get well from one day to the next," was the pronouncement offered to Castorp at the time of his diagnosis.[17] However, Minor gave Frost a more optimistic prognosis. At the time of his discharge in the spring of 1918, Minor wrote to Frost's wife:

> I am shipping back to you this parcel of goods which you seem to value which has been in my care now for the last few months. It is in very good shape, and though there are one or two small rotten spots they are being darned by Nature and I hope will soon be so well that you cannot tell that the goods has been injured. I don't see why Frost should not by fall be able to resume his work. . . .[18]

Discharged by Minor, Frost initially continued his recupera-tion at Exning. He then returned to "light duty" at the Red Cross in Washington. However, a second dread disease was lurking in North America. The great 1918 pandemic of influenza was about to strike. Frost would soon be furiously engaged in the investigation of this epidemic, which would kill more people globally than any previous such firestorm of disease. Light duty was forgotten.

Frost remained active throughout the remainder of his life and had no recurrence of disease. Such an outcome was not unusual for individuals with minimal tuberculosis treated by rest in a sanatorium. The disease of 78 percent of persons admitted to New York State sanatoria with minimal disease remained inactive when followed at fifteen years after their diagnosis; 4 percent had relapsed and 13 percent had died of tuberculosis.[19]

There is another, intriguing construct that one might place on Frost's illness. Perhaps he did not have tuberculosis at all. Frost had spent the preceding four years in Cincinnati, Ohio. Histoplasmosis is a fungal infection of the lungs endemic in the Ohio River valley. The majority of individuals living in that area become infected with *Histoplasma capsulatum*, the causative agent, usually in childhood. Clinical illness is rare, and the infection usually goes unnoticed. Adults moving into the area, as Frost did, are more likely to develop manifest disease, and it commonly mimics pulmonary tuberculosis. In fact, in a survey conducted in the early 1950s many hundreds of patients in tuberculosis sanatoria were actually found to have histoplasmosis. The course of histoplasmosis is usually benign, even when it looks like tuberculosis. Could Frost have had histoplasmosis? The disease was not well understood nor recognized as common in the Cincinnati area until a quarter century after he was given his diagnosis.[20] While such a speculation is interesting, one must remember that tuberculosis struck the Frost family repeatedly. Wade Hampton Frost probably acquired infection with the tubercle bacillus as a child in Marshall.

Whether Frost's disease was or was not tuberculosis, whether his disease was active or inactive, whether his disease was minimal or extensive are not the important questions to address. Rather, it is Frost's perceptions of the "dread disease" that are of consequence. And of this we know or can surmise a good deal. Surely Frost had read Keats under his mother's tutelage. Keats, like Frost, a physician—albeit better known as a poet—had made his own diagnosis after coughing blood. He said to his friend, Charles Brown, "Bring me the candle, Brown, and let me see this blood. . . . That drop of blood is my death warrant; I must die."[21] And from his medical studies Frost would have known of René Theophile Hyacinthe Laennec, the founder of modern pathology and inventor of the stethoscope, who also died of tuberculosis. Furthermore, Frost would also have known of the famous Edward Livingston Trudeau who retreated to Saranac Lake in the Adirondack Mountains of New York and recovered his health, just as had Charles Minor in Asheville. Trudeau, like Keats, dreaded tuberculosis, and when he learned that he was afflicted, he "felt stunned. . . . It meant death and I had never thought of death before! Was I ready to die?"[22] Trudeau practiced for himself, wrote, and taught a doctrine of total withdrawal of tuberculosis patients from normal life's activities. With this dread disease, one must surrender oneself to the malady and retreat to outdoor, preferably mountainous, environs to rest. Cure was never possible, but the person who yielded to tuberculosis might hope for a life of many years as a submissive, chronically ill, but not entirely unhappy patient. These precepts would have been part of Frost's medical curriculum both at the University of Virginia and at Bellevue. In fact, this concept of the management of tuberculosis was the standard of medical care during the first half of the twentieth century.

The "white plague" had become well known to the Frost family. Frost's oldest sister, Mary Deas Frost, had died of tuberculosis in 1904, one year after Frost received his M.D. degree from the University of Virginia. Henry Pinckney Frost, the second Frost child, also developed tuberculosis, but there is no record of the details of his illness or his treatment, and he did not succumb to the disease.[23] Frost's younger brother, Tom, had tuberculosis, first developing the disease some seven years before Wade Hampton Frost himself did and suffering a protracted course. With four of their children thus afflicted, one must ask whether either of the Frost parents had tuberculosis and infected their children. They both lived into older age and appeared to have died of other causes, but that does not mean that they could not have had infectious, but stable and chronic, tuberculosis at earlier times in their lives.

Frost wrote a series of letters to his brother, Tom, about the illness. In two letters written in May of 1922, evidently after his brother had left Asheville before his doctors felt he was ready to return, Frost commented on his brother's discouragement and urged him to return to Asheville. He commented:

> I am near enough kin to you to appreciate very fully (—or so I imagine) just how much and why you hate the idea of all the upset of making "plans" or having them made for you; also how much and why you detest the monotony and discomfort of an indefinite stay in a sanitarium. . . . Nevertheless, . . . I am sure it is worthwhile. . . . Back in 1910, when we first made a diagnosis, I made a mistake for which I have never forgiven myself—the mistake of not *insisting*, against all odds, that you stay in Asheville until Dr. Minor said you were ready to come home.[24]

There is a tone of submission in these letters. That is, Frost clearly believed that the person with tuberculosis must submit to the regimented, confined life of sanatorium care. In *The Magic Mountain* Thomas Mann, whose wife was confined to a sanatorium for the treatment of her tuberculosis, clearly portrays the otherworldliness of sanatorium life. What a conflict this must have presented for Wade Hampton Frost as he contemplated a life with what in those days was considered "arrested," but never cured tuberculosis. In fact, he must have contemplated the possibility that he might spend the rest of his days in a mountain retreat caring for fellow consumptives, as had Trudeau and Minor.

Tom Frost died of the dread disease. In an unfinished letter written on March 15, 1923, the day before his brother's death, Frost wrote:

> There are two factors in the outcome. One, which the doctors can estimate pretty accurately, is the extent of damage to vital organs . . . . The other factor in the case is the less tangible one of "general vitality" or "resistance," and this no doctor can estimate, because it is partly spiritual. . . .[25]

Thoughts of this inestimable "general vitality" must have hounded Wade Hampton Frost throughout his life and as he faced an early death, not from tuberculosis, but cancer. "Vitalism" was a concept of medical etiology popular in the late eighteenth and early nineteenth centuries. It was embraced by Laennec, although he pioneered in "organicism," the belief that alterations in body organs were responsible for disease. By vitalism Laennec and his colleagues meant that some diseases were not caused by organic changes but by alterations in an undefined vital spirit—vitality.[26] This notion of disease etiology persisted in medical thought not as a causation of disease but as a determinant of one's bodily resistance to disease, and clearly Frost viewed his brother's and his own illnesses in those terms. Although Frost had no further episodes of tuberculous disease, that illness was never far from his mind. It served as the focal point for a number of his most important research studies, which occupied much of the last decade of his life. It may also have dictated a structuring, perhaps regimentation, of his daily life, and perhaps contributed to his love of the formalized, mathematical aspects of epidemiology.

Dickens may have had only tuberculosis in mind when he spoke of a "dread disease," but the term certainly should also be applied to influenza as it swept the globe in 1918 and 1919. The "Spanish Flu," as it quickly became called, struck more than a quarter of all Americans and killed more than a half million, more than five times the number killed in World War I. It swept the globe within about six months, and worldwide it may have killed as many as fifty million persons.[27] Both attack rates and death rates were much higher than previous outbreaks of "flu." Most of the deaths occurred in young adults. The military forces on both sides of the European battlefield were so severely hit that it is likely the epidemic had a major role in bringing an end to the fighting. People were said to have dropped dead on city streets, and public panic accompanied the rapid march of this dread disease.[28] In order to properly emphasize the enormous sweep of such a global epidemic, epidemiologists use the term pandemic, a word first coined by William Harvey in 1666.

The influenza virus is a changeable beast. First of all, there are two major types, called A and B. Influenza A is the villain that causes the respiratory illness we all know as flu and that causes epidemics from time to time. Influenza B causes a milder disease and rarely produces epidemics. On its surface influenza A has two proteins that serve as the major antigens recognized by the immunological defense mechanisms of infected persons. These two proteins, hemagglutinin and neuraminidase, are variable in their form, and as they vary so they elude recognition by host defender cells. Virologists simply number the known variants in these proteins. The virus causing the 1918 pandemic is now thought to have been an H1N1 type.[29] The Asian flu virus that struck the United States in 1957 was a H2N2 strain. The virus circulating in North America during the mild influenza season of 2002–2003 was an H3N2 strain. When a mutation or change in one of these surface proteins occurs, an outbreak of flu can be expected. To confuse the picture further, minor changes in the virus also occur— so-called genetic drift—so that one year's type may vary a good bit from that of the next year, even without changes in the major H and N types. That is why flu vaccines must be reformulated each year.

Most new strains of flu virus are thought to arise by mutation and species-hopping of swine and poultry viruses. In modern times, most flu epidemics have started in Asia and then spread globally, presumably because in many parts of Asia people live in relatively close contact with swine and poultry. But that's not what happened in 1918. That epidemic began in the United States.

Thousands and thousands of young American men swarmed into military encampments to train and prepare to join General Pershing in France to fight the "war to end all wars" against the "Huns." The crowded conditions in these camps provided ideal incubators for infectious diseases, as Frost had presciently noted in his earlier memo on the role of the Red Cross in wartime. It was in these military camps that Spanish flu made its debut. On March 11, 1918, influenza struck Fort Riley, Kansas; on March 18 Fort Oglethorpe, Tennessee.[30] The disease spread among military personnel with outbreaks in many army camps. Not surprisingly, the flu spread to nearby communities, again as foreseen by Frost. On March 30, 1918, eighteen cases of severe influenza with three deaths were reported from Haskell, Kansas. About the same time, the Ford Motor Company in Detroit, Michigan, was forced to send home more than a thousand workers who were ill with flu.[31] Somehow, those first outbreaks attracted little public attention. The Public Health Service noted the problem, however, and organized an Office of Field Investigations of Influenza with Wade Hampton Frost, only recently returned from Asheville, pulled from his Red Cross assignment and placed in charge. In a letter to Rupert Blue, Surgeon General, Frost wrote on April 18:

> In compliance with your letter of April 16th, I have the honor to submit herewith a list of the personnel employed in FIELD INVESTI-GATIONS OF INFLUENZA. . . . [The] list also contains names of those employed in Baltimore, Md., Topeka, Kansas, and Boston, Mass.[32]

Frost's list included the names of twenty-eight persons working on the burgeoning epidemic.

Among the group assembled by Frost was Edgar Sydenstricker, a statistician whom Frost first met in this context and who would become an important and trusted colleague and a close friend. Sydenstricker grew up in China; he was the brother of the famous novelist Pearl Sydenstricker Buck. One year younger than Frost, he had joined the Public Health Service only three years previously. He was working with Joseph Goldberger on a Hygienic Laboratory study of pellagra, a nutritional deficiency disease, among South Carolina textile mill workers when he was summoned to join the influenza team. The pellagra study was noteworthy because, among other things, it included house-to-house surveys in an attempt to identify all affected individuals. They were the first such surveys in the field of public health.[33] Household surveys would become part of the influenza investigation and would be featured in later collaborative studies between Frost and

Sydenstricker. In 1919, Sydenstricker was made the Chief Statistician of the Public Health Service. He was stationed in Washington, close enough to Baltimore to facilitate an ongoing collaboration between the two friends during the years while Frost was on the faculty at Johns Hopkins University.

In late August and September the Spanish flu struck Boston and nearby Camp Devens. Medical facilities were quickly overwhelmed. Two of the nation's greatest microbiologists and experts on pneumonias, William Henry Welch of Johns Hopkins University and Oswald T. Avery of the Rockefeller Institute, were called upon by the army to visit Camp Devens. There was little then that could be done for those afflicted beyond supporting them as the illness ran its course. One after another the major cities of America's east coast were attacked. By October, the Public Health Service reported that

> Influenza has spread practically over the entire United States. The greatest numbers of cases are still reported from the Eastern States, but the number in the West is rapidly increasing.[34]

On October 1, 1918, the United States Congress acted to provide resources for the Public Health Service efforts:

> *Resolved*, That to enable the Public Health Service to combat and suppress "Spanish influenza" and other communicable diseases . . . there is appropriated . . . $1,000,000.[35]

A volunteer corps of reserve public health service officers was created and doctors enlisted from communities across America to assist local health departments. Indeed, providing assistance to local health departments was the major focus of most of the national effort.

Troop ships carried the disease to Europe. Brest, a principal port of debarkation for American soldiers in France, was hard hit, and the epidemic then spread across Europe and the globe. Among American troops at home, the attack rate was 36 percent; among naval personnel, 40 percent; among American soldiers in Europe, 17 percent.[36] Armies in the field simply bogged down, unable to function in the face of widespread debilitating illness.

While public health personnel throughout the country issued warnings and advice to a frightened populace, Frost and his coworkers set about the task of determining what was really happening. Weekly reports published in Public Health Reports gave data on influenza outbreaks in various localities, but a broader look would require a more distant perspective. That look was the task undertaken by Frost and his colleagues. And time would have to pass to allow for the picture to be seen in its entirety. In November 1918 a special office was established for this purpose, initially and temporarily located in Baltimore. By January 1919 it was more permanently situated in Washington.[37] Frost and Sydenstricker worked largely alone and together, surrounded by data reports and with the support of eleven clerks and stenographers with their tabulating machines and typewriters. Several other public health officers were assigned to the work for short periods of time.

By the summer of 1919, the pandemic had waned, but the epidemiologic efforts of Frost's team had not. In June Frost and Sydenstricker published a chronology of the global spread of influenza.[38] Three waves had occurred, more or less in synchrony in sites as far separated as Manchester, England, and Bombay, India. They peaked in July 1918, October through December 1918, and February and March 1919.

In August 1919 Frost published a seminal analysis of influenza incidence data. He began by noting the principal problem confronting public health officials seeking to deal with influenza:

> During great epidemics [of influenza] there are abundant, if not exact, records of prevalence, and the resulting mortality can be determined with fair precision, even though a large proportion of the deaths are classified under diagnoses other than influenza. In the intervals between epidemics influenza becomes inextricably confused with other respiratory diseases, having a general clinical resemblance but no definite etiological entity, so that the record of prevalence and even of mortality is virtually lost. The first requisites for epidemiological study, namely, clear differential diagnosis and systematic records of occurrence, are therefore lacking in influenza.
>
> In the absence of these essential records, statistics of mortality from the group comprising influenza and all forms of pneumonia afford,

perhaps, the nearest approximation to a record of influenza. It is not intended to suggest that the mortality from this group of diseases furnishes in any sense a *measure* of the prevalence of influenza, but only that it furnishes an *index*, since it is well established that the epidemic prevalence of influenza markedly affects the mortality from this group of diseases, and since it is at least probable that even in nonepidemic periods there may be some intimate and constant relation between the prevalence of influenza and the mortality from pneumonia.[39]

Frost then carefully tabulated and graphed the pneumonia and influenza data from Massachusetts, one of the only states for which such data were available, for the years 1887 through 1916. His chart of these data is presented in figure 7.1. This chart demonstrated

the effect of the epidemic of 1889–1892, developing in three distinct phases; the first culminating in January 1890, the second in April and May 1891, and the third in January 1892. It is noted that the mortality was higher in 1891 than in 1890, still higher in 1892; and that in 1893, although no distinct epidemic occurred, the pneumonia mortality for the year was still higher than in 1892.[40]

Frost continued his analysis by examining the pneumonia and influenza death rates for 1910 through 1918 in Cleveland, San Francisco, and New York City. Again, he observed a close correlation. Moreover, he noted, the recent influenza epidemic had been associated with an unusually high death rate. The importance of this paper lies in Frost's observation and careful documentation of the correlation between epidemic influenza, for which concurrently reported public health data are not generally available, and pneumonia deaths, which can be readily documented from death certificates. For decades thereafter, excess mortality from respiratory illness was used to track the course of influenza epidemics. Today, sentinel clinics in selected North American cities collect data and perform viral cultures of individuals thought to be suffering from influenza. The predominant circulating strain is established each year in time for vaccine manufacturers to prepare vaccine. But warnings to Americans that an unusually severe epidemic may be

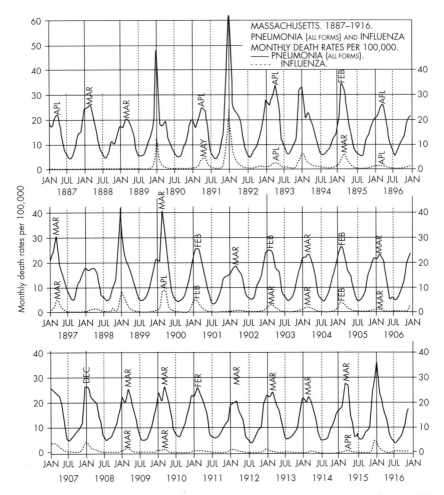

Figure 7.1. Pneumonia and influenza mortality for Massachusetts from 1887 to 1916 as charted by Frost and demonstrating correlation between deaths due to the two diseases in epidemic years. See text for Frost's discussion of this figure. Reproduced from Frost WH. The epidemiology of influenza. *Public Health Rep.* 1919; 34:1823–36.

upon them are still the product of Frostian analyses of pneumonia deaths.

In February 1920, Sydenstricker and Mary L. King published a discussion of some of the statistical difficulties facing those who wished to obtain an accurate picture of the magnitude of the influenza epidemic.[41] They noted that four million men in

the age group most afflicted in this epidemic had been with-
drawn from the general population to enter the military services. This had a substantial effect on the denominators of
population size used in computing community incidences and
prevalences. Thoughtful considerations of this type would
become a hallmark of Frost's future epidemiological work.
Sydenstricker, with whom he continued to collaborate, probably had an important influence upon his thinking in this
regard.

Frost's last major work on the influenza epidemic was an
attempt to get around the problems of dealing with a disease
for which there was no reporting system in place, by conducting house-to-house surveys in selected communities. The influence of Sydenstricker is apparent in this study. It is also
reminiscent of Frost's early experience with "shoe-leather epidemiology," investigating outbreaks of typhoid fever and
polio. While limited to sample communities, data of this type
provided the opportunity for a more detailed look at the disease than did case and death reports. An initial survey was
conducted in several communities in Maryland.[42] This was
followed by the canvassing by trained investigators of nine
other communities selected to be broadly representative of the
United States.[43] As seen in figure 7.2, the age-specific influenza
mortality data produced a curve reminiscent of the two-humped
back of a Bactrian camel. The deaths in older individuals were
not unexpected; the peak in young adults was a surprise that
characterized this outbreak. Again noted in this survey-based
study was the correlation between influenza rates and deaths
due to all forms of respiratory disease.

During the years devoted to influenza, Frost and his family
lived in the Toronto Apartments at Twentieth and P Streets
near Dupont Circle in Washington, D.C. Washington and the
Dupont Circle area were familiar territory to the couple, especially to Susan, who had lived there for roughly a decade
before meeting Frost. The influenza epidemic had passed, but
Frost and his colleagues were busy for some time with the
large amount of data they had collected. In fact, Frost's interest
in influenza continued into later years when some of his

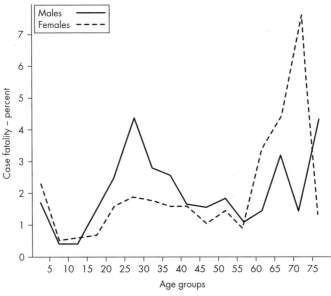

Influenza–case fatality (per cent) in males and females of each specified
age group in all localities canvassed

Figure 7.2. Age-specific mortality data for the 1918–1919 influenza epidemic
collected during surveys in selected American communities. Note the peaks
of mortality in both older and young adult age groups. Reproduced from
Frost WH. Statistics of influenza morbidity. With special reference to certain
factors in case incidence and case fatality. *Public Health Rep.* 1920; 35:584–97.

research focused on the epidemiology of a number of acute
respiratory infections. In 1930 he joined a group of Public
Health Service statisticians, including Sydenstricker, in analyz-
ing influenza data for the period 1910 to 1929.[44] Nominally
Frost would again be in charge of the reopened Cincinnati-
based water investigations, to which he was reassigned on
September 26, 1919. He returned only for brief intervals to
Cincinnati, however. Other things were on his mind.

8

Baltimore

It was grand to have you here. . . . Most of the
time [was] spent talking not about ourselves, but
in letting conversation just ripple along.
—Wade Hampton Frost[1]

Following the conclusion of World War I and under the leadership of William Welch, Johns Hopkins University opened its School of Hygiene and Public Health, the first such institution in the United States. Wade Hampton Frost became its first professor of epidemiology.

Johns Hopkins was a wealthy, unmarried, Quaker, Baltimore businessman who viewed his wealth as carrying an obligation to serve humanity. He established and endowed corporations for Johns Hopkins University and Johns Hopkins Hospital, each with twelve directors (ten individuals served on both boards). To each he gave $3.5 million in 1867. From the start, he indicated that medical education was to be an important function of the university. Although his endowment did not specifically link the hospital to the university, there was never doubt in the minds of the trustees that they should be tightly associated.[2]

William Henry Welch was a Connecticut Yankee, born in Norfolk, Connecticut, on April 8, 1850. He attended Yale University, where he studied the classics, a field in which he hoped to make his career as an academician. Failing to gain a faculty appointment, he studied chemistry at Yale and then medicine at the College of Physicians and Surgeons in New York City. After an internship at Bellevue Hospital in the same city, he joined the hospital's department of pathology. Exciting things in medicine were taking place in Europe, and soon Welch was in Germany, where he spent two years and learned the techniques of the new discipline of bacteriology. He returned to New York and promptly became one of America's preeminent bacteriologists. He established the first American course in that science. His reputation grew, and he was recruited to Johns Hopkins in 1885 as chairman of the department of pathology. From that post, he went on to become dean of the medical school and then acting president of the university.[3] But he did not forget bacteriology, and he kept in his mind the idea of a separate institute or school that would contribute knowledge to the understanding of infectious diseases and the health problems related to them. He remembered the institutes of hygiene that had emerged in Germany and at which he had studied.

"Popsy" Welch had a profound impact on American medicine and medical education. He was described by a student as follows:

> [He] was a short man, only a few inches over five feet tall. . . . He was stout but no one thought of him as fat. . . . His face was not handsome. It was pink and human and good-natured. His eyes were small and blue and deeply set. His mouth was not large, but the lips were full, almost feminine. His chin was hidden by a not too closely clipped beard.[4]

In 1917 with world war raging, Welch, then sixty-seven years old, joined the army as a medical officer. His duties were largely ceremonial, chiefly consisting of visiting military installations to review their sanitary conditions. Following the war he returned to Johns Hopkins and turned his attention to establishing a facility for public health at that university. The Rockefeller Foundation was prepared to fund a school of public health—there were none in North America at that time—and a great deal of political infighting ensued between leaders in the field in New York, at Yale, and at Harvard. Welch argued for more than a school to train sanitarians. He sought an institution on the model of German institutes of hygiene that would teach the disciplines underlying public health and that would function as an institute to conduct research relevant to those disciplines. His view prevailed, and thus, on June 12,

1916, the Executive Committee of the Rockefeller Foundation awarded Johns Hopkins University $267,000 to establish the School of Hygiene and Public Health at Johns Hopkins University.

For the next several years, the foundation provided operating expenses, originally projected to be $50,000 annually, but seemingly increasing without end. Welch was the school's director, and William H. Howell was recruited from the Johns Hopkins School of Medicine department of physiology to be the first professor at the new school, chair of the department of physiological hygiene, and the school's assistant director. Howell assumed most of the administrative functions of the directorship from the start, and he became director in 1926. In 1922, the Rockefeller Foundation, facing ever-increasing demands for additional grants, awarded $6 million to the school, including $1 million for the construction of a new building and $5 million to provide a permanent endowment, the income from which would support operating expenses. Thereafter, the foundation indicated, the school could no longer expect that it would pick up financial short-falls.

The first class, with eight students, was admitted on October 1, 1918. Initially classes were held in buildings left vacant when the undergraduate university had moved to a new campus. In October 1926 the new building at 615 North Wolfe Street, which was to become the permanent home of the school, was opened.[5] This building is still in use, although it has been remodeled and enlarged by additions to each side and the back. It is shown in figure 8.1 as it appeared at the time it opened.

William Welch had a legendary eye for academic medical talent, and he soon identified Wade Hampton Frost as his choice for the first faculty post in epidemiology. Frost was winding down his influenza activities when Welch approached him early in the summer of 1919. In fact, the Public Health Service assigned him to Washington on July 24, 1919, and placed him in charge of morbidity statistics for the service, with Edgar Sydenstricker and Dean K. Brundage assisting him as

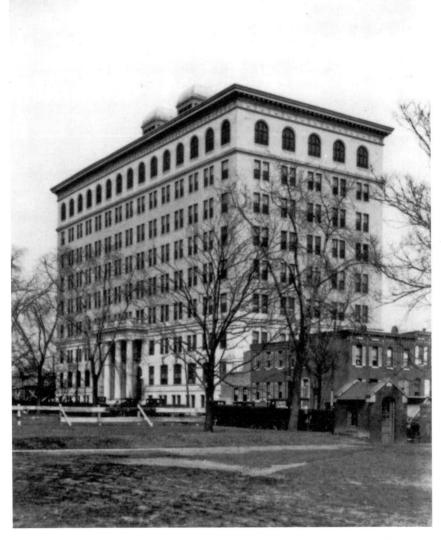

Figure 8.1. The Johns Hopkins School of Hygiene and Public Health building at 615 North Wolfe Street as it appeared at the time of its completion in 1926. Photograph is from the Alan Mason Chesney Archives of the Medical Institutions of the Johns Hopkins University. Reproduced with permission.

statisticians. Rupert Blue was the Surgeon General of the Public Health Service at that time (he was succeeded by Frost's personal friend, Hugh Cumming, on March 3, 1920), and even before Frost's assignment to the statistics post, Welch had

contacted Blue to discuss the possibility of a temporary assignment to Johns Hopkins. Welch invited Frost to Baltimore, and
Frost soon found himself excited by the prospect of moving to
the academic environment of the new school. The discussions
dragged on, however, and Frost, who was not accustomed to
delays in negotiations, became impatient. On July 18, 1919, he
wrote to Welch, cautiously saying that he was "rather anxious
to get on with my plans."[6] He was soon to travel to Cincinnati
to reorganize the reopened station there, and, he said, "I can
hardly establish any definite organization there until I know
what my own status is going to be." Also, he noted, his lease
on his Washington apartment would soon have to be renewed
if he were to stay in that city. Blue agreed to the assignment,
and Frost's Public Health Service duty station became Johns
Hopkins University in Baltimore, Maryland, on September 16,
1919. Officially, he was "on loan" to the university as a result
of the arrangement negotiated between Welch and Blue.[7] His
academic appointment was as a resident lecturer. Welch
charged him with creating a curriculum and a department of
epidemiology.

In 1922, then Surgeon General Hugh Cumming asked Frost
whether he would be willing to leave Johns Hopkins to
assume the directorship of a to-be-created division of scientific
research of the Public Health Service. Frost replied tactfully
that he wished to continue his Public Health Service work on
stream pollution while remaining at Johns Hopkins. However,
he acknowledged, "I have been forced to the conclusion that
the present arrangement, agreeable as it is to me in many
respects, is unsatisfactory from the standpoint of both the
Service and of the School."[8] In the summer of 1929, Frost told
Cumming, by then a good personal friend, that he intended to
resign his commission, which he did effective as of August 8,
1929. He was given a reserve commission and continued to
function as a consultant to the Public Health Service in the area
of water pollution.

The Frost family—Susie was now three—moved to Baltimore in
the fall of 1919. Baltimore's residential areas are famous for red

brick row houses with white marble steps, all set one against another. The Frosts found housing on Lanvale Street in just such a neighborhood. Theirs was not a row house, however. They rented a small English cottage-style house in which they lived during their first two years in Baltimore. William Howell lived just down the street. Howell quickly made friends with the Frosts, especially with Susan.

Situated on the Patapsco River near its entry into Chesapeake Bay, Baltimore had a superb deep water harbor, and its early history depended in large part upon its role as a port. The harbor was guarded by Fort McHenry, above which the star spangled banner immortalized by Francis Scott Key flew in 1814. At the time the Frosts took up residence there, Baltimore was

> a provincial city, a mixture of northern industrialism and southern social attitudes; the School of Hygiene [and Public Health] was the one place in the city where people of many races and cultural backgrounds could meet on grounds of social and intellectual equality.[9]

In the early twentieth century, East Baltimore, which would become important in Frost's academic life, remained an area of manufacturing and activities related to the port. Most of the city's residential areas were located to the north and west, including Roland Park, which was to become the Frosts' neighborhood for many years.

Moving to Baltimore was not, for the Frosts, a venture into the unknown. Rather, it was somewhat of a homecoming. Susan Frost had many relatives in the area. In her daughter's words, "her family seemed to be every other person in Virginia and about half of the population of Baltimore."[10] Susan's sister, Louise Harris, known as Ouida, lived in Baltimore, as did her uncle, J. Triplett Haxall. Carlyle Barton, a cousin, served as a trustee of Johns Hopkins University, although the Frosts had little contact with him. Susan's niece, Emily Randall, would become a social worker at the Harriet Lane Hospital, the Johns Hopkins pediatric unit. Many of these relatives and others lived in the Roland Park neighborhood and became good friends. Susan and Ouida were particularly close.

In 1921, the Frosts moved to live with Ouida, who was ill at the time and for whom Susan wished to provide care and assistance, at 3820 Roland Avenue. After about a year, they took an apartment in the Tudor Hall Apartments at University Parkway and Fortieth Street on the edge of Roland Park. Initially they lived on the fourth floor; later they acquired a large first floor apartment. In 1926 the Frosts purchased their first house at 4710 Keswick Road. A small house, it sat back from the street on a bank and had a porch across the front. Neighbors' houses crowded close to it on each side. The Frosts made this house their home for nearly a decade. In 1935 they purchased a large house at 508 Woodlawn Road. This dwelling had at one time been a boarding house. Real estate sales were sluggish during the depression years of the 1930s, and the Woodlawn house had been on the market for some time and was in poor repair. The Frosts set about making it their home. Figure 8.2 shows this dwelling with its large porch across the front and along one side. The house had sufficient space to provide a separate study for Frost as well as a guest room for visitors. It had three bathrooms, and a large kitchen—the domain of Eva Anderson. Frost was not destined to live for more than a few years thereafter, but Susan stayed on in that house, often with relatives as boarders, until 1958, when a disabling stroke forced her to move to a more manageable situation in a near-by apartment building.[11] The Roland Park neighborhood, where Frost and many of his faculty colleagues lived, was about six or seven miles from the East Baltimore location of the School of Hygiene and Public Health, about a thirty-minute drive through the city. Roland Park remains to this day a gracious and attractive residential neighborhood, described by one Baltimorean as one of "old money."[12]

Eva Anderson, who had worked for the Frosts since early in their marriage, continued to live with and serve the Frost family. She was very much a part of the family, and she was in many ways a surrogate mother for the daughter. Eva Jane Bridget Anderson was born in the Free State area near Marshall, Virginia, on December 28, 1896. Henry Frost had delivered her and provided medical care for her and her nine

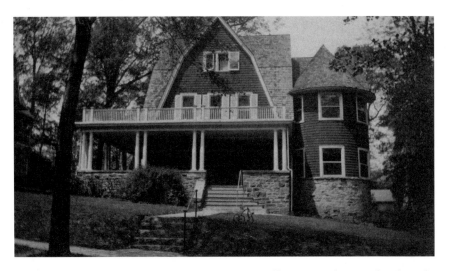

Figure 8.2. The Frost residence at 508 Woodlawn Road in Roland Park, Baltimore. Photograph is from the Claude Moore Health Sciences Library, University of Virginia Health Sciences Center, Charlottesville, VA: Wade Hampton Frost Archives, Box 7, Folder 12. Reproduced with permission, courtesy of the Historical Collection and Services of the Claude Moore Health Sciences Library.

siblings. Harriet Frost had taught her to read and write. Having worked for the senior Frosts, she went to Exning after their deaths to assist Susan, who had moved there from Cincinnati with her infant daughter after her automobile accident. Eva Anderson was seventeen years old at that time. Often referred to as the cook, she was indeed an excellent cook (she learned most of her recipes from Susan Frost), but in fact, Anderson was much more than a cook. She was housekeeper, baby sitter, and often practical nurse. She was estranged from her much older husband—who was the Frosts' furnace man—and would have nothing to do with him. Anderson had a good sense of humor. She was well known to most of the Frost's friends, and they stopped in the kitchen to enjoy her animated and often satirical wit. Her kitchen was frequently crowded with neighborhood children listening to her stories. Her twins, Mary Jane and Billy, commonly called "the Frost twins," were also a regular part of the household.[13]

When the Frosts put apartment living behind them and became home owners on Keswick Road, Susan took up gardening with great enthusiasm. Occasionally she hired a handyman to do some of the heavy spading, but for the most part she did all of the work herself. Eva Anderson, who was held in great respect in the family for her "green thumb," joined Susan in the garden. Eventually, Susan interested her husband in her gardens, and Frost also became a digger in the dirt and an enthusiast for the garden. In fact, he filled a sun room in the house with seedlings that he had started. He crowded the tender plants too closely in their flats, and he ignored Anderson's sage advice to thin them.[14]

The Woodlawn Road house was infested with termites, and Frost resisted his wife's effort to summon an exterminator. Instead, he consulted an entomologist from the Johns Hopkins faculty. The two men crawled around the house, but their efforts were unsuccessful. Ultimately, Susan prevailed and the termites were successfully banished.[15]

Pets were regular additions to the Frost household. The family had a series of cats. Millie, who joined the family at Exning about the time Frost returned from Asheville, had many kittens, requiring some effort to arrange for their disposition. During the time the Frosts lived on the fourth floor of the Tudor Hall Apartments, Lucy, one of Millie's kittens, fell down a gutter drain pipe. With squeals and howls emanating from both Millie and Lucy, Susan called to Lucy, "Lucy, Lucy, we're coming," to try to reassure the trapped kitten while her husband went to a neighbor's home to borrow tools to cut the pipe and liberate the animal.

Cats were not the only pets. Looper, a dog at the Lanvale Street home, was most notable for its habit of chewing shoes. As time went on, Bobo, an Airedale, joined the family as did Polly, a parrot, and Nutty, a squirrel that was frequently fed peanut brittle. Bobo was a wanderer and would not stay home, so Susan returned him to her aunt, Elsie Barton, who had given the dog to her. Daughter Susan had a pet cat named Brownie when she was eight or ten years old. Brownie slept with the girl, curled up under the sheets of the bed at her feet. When

Brownie was killed by a dog, Frost left his office in the middle of the day in response to his wife's call—an unprecedented action—to tell his daughter about the death of her pet.[16]

The Keswick Road house—and indeed the later house on Woodlawn Road—was inhabited by bats. On seeing a bat, Susan Frost would scream and cover her head with a sheet. Typically, the dog would chase the bat, on one occasion jumping on the hot stove in its pursuit, while Frost tried to deal with the intruder. One time, while Dr. Lewis R. (Jimmy) and Mabel Thompson were house guests, the two doctors went after a bat with a broom and a paper bag in which they hoped to confine the bat. Frost tripped on a blanket chest mounted on caster wheels and caromed down the hall.[17]

The Frosts entertained frequently, sometimes other faculty members, sometimes foreign visitors, sometimes students. They often housed distinguished visitors in their home, displacing their daughter to a bed in the hall or the attic to turn her bedroom into a guest room. In the large Woodlawn Road house, they had a guest bedroom, which was frequently occupied. The Frosts were gifted hosts. Baltimore was close enough to Washington to allow their circle of friends to extend to the nation's capital.

Reflecting on international visitors to their home, Frost's daughter recalled:

> A hot summer day. But WHF (with me as passenger, as he was then the only driver in the family) drove his '29 Ford across town . . . to pick up [Dr. Garrido Morales and his wife, who were visiting from Puerto Rico] for a drive in the countryside and tea, or a meal, at our house. And drove them back.[18]

Hugh de Valin, a Public Health Service officer with whom Frost had worked during the New Orleans yellow fever epidemic, always made a point of visiting the Frosts and often stayed with them whenever he was in the Washington area. He and Eva Anderson enjoyed a bantering relationship. Laura Carter was a frequent visitor and house guest. Her father, army colonel Henry Rose Carter, had done much to elucidate the epidemiology and pathogenesis of yellow fever. Frost had known and admired him, and had served as a pall bearer at his funeral. Carter had left an unfinished tome on yellow fever, which his daughter was trying to edit and prepare for publication, and Frost helped her with this project. Laura Carter and Susan Frost became good friends.

English colleagues were guests on visits to Johns Hopkins. Among them, Sir Arthur Newsholme and his wife were especially welcome. Newsholme, a distinguished British sanitarian and an early investigator of the epidemiology of tuberculosis, was nearing the end of his academic career in England. He had been brought from London by Welch to teach public health administration. Because it interested him, he included epidemiology in his teaching at the new school. After Frost arrived and assumed responsibility for that subject, Newsholme returned at intervals as a guest lecturer. Newsholme and Frost became friends, and from time to time they taught classes in epidemiology jointly. The Newsholmes were not the only British guests. On one occasion, Sir Wilson Jameson and George Auden visited the Frost home for tea and set about demonstrating to Susan and Eva Anderson the proper English way to brew tea. Their product did not pass muster; the American water was the problem, of course.[19]

Susan, usually called Sue by her friends, enjoyed the role of faculty wife and the attendant hostess duties. Their daughter later recalled:

> I've heard it said of my mother many times that she could walk into a room full of people who were ill at ease or very shy and in very short order put them at ease. . . . As a matter of fact, . . . my father did the same thing. At a very tense gathering, he instantly—just in his very quiet way—saw what the situation was and smoothed everything over. . . . My mother you might have called a "social animal," . . . although my father enjoyed people no less and was awfully good with them. [Ours] was a very socially busy household, . . . but in a very casual, quiet way.[20]

Among the social duties readily accepted by Susan Frost was the entertainment of students. Many of them were from other countries, often newly arrived in Baltimore to pursue the public health studies. Some of them held positions of substantial academic, political, and social importance in their own countries, but most of them were intimidated by life in America. Welch had established a social organization to support them, which he named the "Ubiquiteers." Later this club became elitist with highly sought election to membership, and the school changed it to include all students. As remembered by Susan Frost Parrish:

> At least annually . . . my parents gave [teas] for the students at the School of Hygiene. I'm afraid that for many it may have been about the only time that they were invited to an American household— some of the foreign students. These were not formal affairs, although they probably seemed so to the students.[21]

Formal or not in the memory of their daughter, the Frosts always dressed up for these teas.

On some occasions, entertainment was considerably more formal. William Howell and Susan Frost shared a common birthday, and it was always celebrated with a dinner at the Frost home. With twelve to fourteen guests drawn from the roster of Johns Hopkins faculty colleagues seated around the dining table, there were many toasts. Some guests wrote bits of verse for the occasion; Susan was remembered by her daughter as especially clever at writing poetry for such events. Of course, not all of the formal dinners were free of amusing moments, sometimes unexpected. On one occasion while they were living at the Tudor Hall apartment, Charles, a butler hired to serve at a fancy dinner party, was drunk and spilled French dressing down a lady guest's dress.

On other, less pretentious occasions, humor was much a part of the evening's program, and sometimes practical jokes as well. Susan Frost Parrish later reflected on her mother:

> My mother in particular had one of the keenest senses of the ridiculous that I have ever encountered. She could really roll them in the aisles. There was so much laughter. . . . This is part of what made the era so agreeable.[22]

At one evening meal Susan Frost, with the collusion of Eva Anderson, served George Ramsey, Jack Frost's exceptionally shy, bachelor, junior faculty member, a rubber hot dog. Ramsey had declined the meat being served, and when Susan asked him what he would prefer, he replied that he was very fond of hot dogs, assuming that it would take little effort to produce one for him. Out came the rubber sausage adorned with parsley. Ramsey tried to cut it, with great embarrassment followed by hilarity.[23]

Frost was a quiet person in the presence of his talkative wife, who usually dominated conversations with visitors. A modest, gentle person, he was considered shy only by those who did not know him well. His wife's nephew, Marshall Barton, described him as "diffident."

> He was [a person] who really, I think, disliked "small talk," but he enjoyed talking about something of substance.[24]

At that time, "something of substance" often meant the mounting threat of war as reported on a daily basis in the newspapers. Frost was particularly upset by what he considered flawed reasoning in analyzing the events abroad. He expected the same rigor in newspaper reporting that he required of himself in his professional life. Again, in the words of Barton:

> He was always on the alert for logical fallacies that he could detect in the work of others. . . . Without being tedious about it, . . . he [periodically] expressed annoyance at sloppy reasoning he would see stated in the papers. . . . It was a very parlous time. This was Hitler building up towards the Second World War and everything. We thought we saw stupidities going on all over the place, in this country as well as Europe.[25]

Parlous times they were, and Frost was greatly worried about the failures of the League of Nations, Mussolini's incursions into Ethiopia and the horn of Africa, and Hitler's ascendency in Germany. In January 1938, Frost, then ill with cancer, wrote to his daughter:

> I think what really has me "down" . . . is my profound discouragement over the state of the world. . . . Not in one country alone, but throughout the world, men are more and more heading in the direction of disaster. . . . I am not sure what lies ahead, but it must be a fight.[26]

Among the logical fallacies Frost perceived were the increasingly popular ideas of Sigmund Freud. In a letter to his daughter he wrote:

> His ideas, tho' discredited by the most scientific of psychologists & psychiatrists . . . are still very popular with the rank and file of psychologists & with fiction-writers. . . . I tell you that someone who has great fame as a scientist is actually "talking through his hat" & doing more harm than good.[27]

As suggested by these remarks, Frost was somewhat prudish in a Victorian way. In that letter he commented on a book he had observed in his married daughter's possession, apparently a book about sex and reproduction.

> What an intelligent well-educated person needs to know of the reproductive process is not much beyond a few simple facts of anatomy and physiology, such as are given in any good college text on physiology. Beyond this there are some things that are learned and are intended to be learned only by each person's own experience. . . . For what is essential to know and feel about the sex-relation is so vital to the human race that Nature takes no chances with poor teachers. She makes it a matter of *instinct*.[28]

Frost was interested in politics and current events. Foreign affairs were also frequently on his mind, perhaps stimulated by the contact with many foreign students at Johns Hopkins. Susan shared these interests, and the news of the day was a frequent topic of conversation in the Frost home, with or without guests present. The Frosts paid attention to the daily newspapers; John Owens, the editor of the *Baltimore Sun*, was a close friend. They listened to radio broadcasts only occasionally.

Despite his strong religious upbringing in Marsall, Frost never attended church. Nominally Episcopalians, the Frosts sent their daughter to Sunday school. They themselves stayed home, not so much out of disagreement with their religion as a feeling that it was not relevant to their lives. Spiritual matters did not find a place on the Frost intellectual agenda.

The Frosts were liberals and supporters of Roosevelt's New Deal. When asked about her father's feelings towards FDR, his daughter recalled:

Oh, he was very strongly for him in the beginning. . . . My father was certainly an internationalist. . . . I honestly don't know whether he was a registered Democrat, but . . . both he and my mother thought that way. I do remember very well how strongly they felt about the huge businesses—what we now call corporate businesses—putting small businessmen out of work. Specifically, I remember a conversation about the Rockefellers' swallowing of the smaller companies. . . . I think the label "Jeffersonian Democrat," for whatever that means, [might be] the proper one. . . . This would have . . . some shadings of economic conservatism in it. . . . I think he was concerned about a very strong concentration of power in the government. Well, the answer is, yes, I think he admired a great deal of that [which] Roosevelt set out to do.[29]

Frost was a supporter of prepaid health insurance, a radical idea at the time. "I have long been an advocate of sickness insurance, in part compulsory; and that, I think, is the opinion of nearly all serious students of the subjects," he wrote to his daughter, who was then working in Boston, in 1937.[30]

The Frosts were always surrounded by books. Both of them were avid readers. Presents of books were particularly welcomed by the bibliophiles and often received from friends or relatives. Susan Frost had a set of bookplates depicting the Frost family crest made by a London engraver, but her husband thought them pretentious and never used them. Frost had been schooled in the classics, including Latin and Greek, by his mother, and he found great pleasure in reading the works of Roman masters in the original Latin. Harking back to his South Carolina roots, he was interested in the Gullah culture of that state's coastal tidewater area, and he enjoyed Edwin DuBose Heyward's *Porgy*, the story upon which George Gershwin based his opera, *Porgy and Bess*. Susan joined him in this interest.[31]

"Jack" Frost was a serious scholar and also a fun-loving man. He occasionally joined a group that met on Saturday evenings at Schellhase's, a Baltimore speak-easy and restaurant at 412 North Howard Street, for conversation, music, and bootleg German beer. H. L. Mencken, the iconoclastic editor, writer, and satirical social critic, was a gourmet, a pianist, and the organizer of what came to be known as the "Saturday Night Club."

The group, of which Frost was not a formal member, met for dinner in a back room and drank beer from glass mugs engraved with their names or, as visitors, from mugs denominated "Deadhead." Many of Baltimore's professional and literary notables attended, and one can presume that the conversation was not limited to discussion of the quality of the beer.[32] Frost did not like Mencken as a person. However, the two men did have lively conversations, and Frost, who was himself a meticulous craftsman of written English, respected and admired Mencken's usage of the language in his writings. In the mind of Marshall Barton, Susan Frost's nephew who lived with the Frosts in the Woodlawn Road house for about two years while in law school, Frost "was kind of amused by Mencken and outraged by Mencken a little bit. I don't think he was very pro-Mencken too much, although it was very hard to be neutral."[33]

Frost probably attended sessions of the "Saturday Night Club" as the guest of his faculty colleague, Raymond Pearl. Pearl, who headed the department of biostatistics, was a member and regular participant in the meetings of the club; he played the French horn with the group. Frost had easy relationships with Pearl, as he did with all of his professional colleagues, and the Pearls lived close to the Frosts. Yet the two families were not particularly close. Pearl was an outspoken and aggressive man whose personality differed greatly from that of Frost. Susan Frost did not like Pearl.

Mencken was a notorious critic of the South and its traditions. When Barton was asked whether he recalled Frost as having strong feelings about the South, he mused:

> Well, he was from the South. . . . [However,] I would say he wasn't fighting the war, at all, but [he] found it a fascinating subject . . . and of course, knew an awful lot about it and remembered the battles and turning points and that sort of stuff. . . . No, I would say that his attitude . . . was not anti-North or violently pro-South or anything of that sort, [but] balanced.[34]

Frost had no interest in most sports—baseball, football, and others that filled the pages of back sections of the newspapers.

"We didn't talk about sports," recalled Barton. "He didn't give a damn about sports."[35] The enthusiasm for football he displayed by writing a pep song during his University of Virginia student days had long since waned. But he enjoyed watching horse races and polo matches, perhaps reflecting a boyhood in which a horse or a horse-drawn buggy was the normal mode of transportation. Frost played golf occasionally, using the course at the Elkridge Club a short distance from the Roland Park house in which he lived. "Jimmy" Thompson and Hugh de Valin were his frequent partners on the links.[36] Frost also liked to play bridge. He found it intellectually challenging, and he played the game well.

The Frosts had a wide circle of friends in Baltimore drawn from faculty colleagues, Haxall relatives, and others. Among the faculty colleagues, James A. Doull and his wife were particularly close friends. Doull was an early member of Frost's new department of epidemiology. The Doull's lived on Winslow Road in the Roland Park neighborhood and were frequent vistors to the Frost home. Daughter Susan Frost recalled that the two families "rescued each other's cats and broken down automobiles."[37] Mrs. Doull had a notable singing voice, and she, Rose Haxall Johnson, and Hugh de Valin often provided evening entertainment singing around the Frost's upright Steinway piano.

George Ramsey later joined Frost and Doull on the Johns Hopkins faculty, and he also became a close friend. Edgar Sydenstricker, the Public Health Service statistician with whom Frost had worked so closely, was another frequent visitor to the Frost home. Lowell Reed was recruited to Johns Hopkins by Raymond Pearl and followed him as chairman of the department of biometry and vital statistics. Reed, a gentle man with a quiet wit, developed a close collaboration with Frost and joined him in teaching the mathematical aspects of epidemiology. He and his wife became good friends of Jack and Sue. Alexander (Sandy) Gilliam joined Frost as an associate late in his career, and the two men developed an especially warm relationship. Gilliam was a Virginian and a graduate of that state's university. Frost gave his University of Virginia mortar board to the younger man. Anna Baetjer, a student and later faculty colleague of Frost, and her sister, Ruth, became close friends of Susan.

Lewis R. (Jimmy) Thompson was Jack Frost's occasional golf partner and one of his closest friends. Thompson had conducted field investigations of the polluted Ohio River under Frost in Cincinnati. Thompson joined Frost in investigating the New York City polio epidemic and worked with Frost in preparing the report of that investigation. He was stationed in Washington during many of the years when the Frosts lived in Baltimore, and in 1930 became Assistant Surgeon General and Chief of the Division of Scientific Research for the Public Health Service. In 1937 he became the director of the National Institutes of Health in Bethesda, Maryland.

Ivan M. Marty and his wife, Elizabeth (Betty) Tabb Marty were close friends. Marty worked in the Maryland State Health Department, and came to know Frost professionally. A friendship developed. In the words of Frost's daughter:

> There was a kind of natural affinity, as well as deep affection, between my parents and the Martys. They and [my father] deeply loved simple, country life and the beauty of real countryside. . . . My impression is that the Martys, like my parents, always had a rough going "making ends meet" . . . but out of consideration for others and plain good taste saw to it that one wasn't aware of their being financially strapped.[38]

William Howell and his wife were friends, and so also was William Welch. "Popsy," never married and a gourmet, was formal in all his conduct. He never called Frost either Wade or Jack—always simply "Frost." In later years he did come to use Susan's first name. Frost was one of a very few individuals who was able to say no to Welch. Welch was remembered warmly by daughter Susan Frost Parrish:

> Dr. Welch used to be quite often at the house. I think it bothered my father, but it did not bother my mother to think of asking Dr. Welch to come for the evening. It had nothing to do with professional matters. [My father] was horrified, I remember, at one point when my mother

[and some of her friends] organized a birthday party for [a] Mrs. Weed, [who was] about Dr. Welch's age, at the Hamilton Street Club, the ladies' club. They devised a May pole with streamers, of course, around which Dr. Welch and Mrs. Weed danced along with all the others.

Referring to Welch's presence at the Frost home, Susan Parish continued:

[I remember an occasion—it] must have been a summer occasion, as I can still see him sitting on our porch, characteristically a Roland Park porch, a big one that ran around two sides of the house. Sitting next to [him was] a Chinese lady in full, classical regalia who, as I recall, was the wife of the then Surgeon General of China, whose son was a student at the School of Hygiene. She was wearing long, floor-length robes of satin and silk.[39]

Haxall relatives abounded in Baltimore. Aside from Susan's younger sister, "Ouida" Haxall Harris, Agnes Barton and her husband John (Jack) Duer became good friends, especially of Jack Frost. Duer died at an early age, but his widow remained close to Frost. She had dropped out of school in her teenage years with tuberculosis of the hip and remained a semi-invalid. Highly intelligent, she read avidly and viewed the world with a well-spiced wit. Frost respected her and enjoyed hearing her views.

Salaries were not large at Johns Hopkins University, and money became a problem for many families when the prosperity of the 1920s gave way to the great economic depression of the 1930s. President Herbert Hoover's dream of "a chicken in every pot" was never realized for many Americans. In 1933 salaries at the School of Hygiene and Public Health were cut by 10 percent for senior faculty, 5 percent for the less-well-paid junior faculty and staff members.[40] While the Frosts were not poor, neither were they wealthy. Their Keswick Road home was modest, yet they entertained without stint as they thought appropriate for a university professor. Although, the Frosts weathered the depression without great sacrifice, there were times when it was difficult for them to manage their expenses. Economies were needed, and Susan, who liked to sew, served as seamstress for the house.

She made all of the curtains and slip covers, as she had done previously for their Washington apartment. She also made all of her husband's shirts. In March 1935 Frost resigned from the University Club. "For several years," he wrote, "[I have] felt that continuance of [the] membership . . . was [an] agreeable luxury that would have to be sacrificed." He felt it necessary, in his words, "to lighten ship" by giving up what he enjoyed as "a luxury rather than a necessity."[41] At this time the Frosts had just purchased their large Woodlawn Road house, which probably imposed additional constraints on their budget.

Those of the era who were not in grave financial trouble were concerned about those who were less fortunate, however. Women baked, and Susan and her teenage daughter made trips to Hampden, a blue-collar neighborhood of mill workers, to share the products of the Frost kitchen. Susan opened the first thrift shop in Baltimore, the forerunner of a later such shop at Johns Hopkins known as the "Carry On Shop." This enterprise provided an outlet for unfortunate individuals who were forced to sell possessions in order to put food on the table.[42]

Reflecting some four decades later on her childhood and family life during those difficult years, Susan Frost Parrish commented:

> I look back on [that] era as a special time in terms of spirit or aura. It seems to me that there was, aside from a very interesting mix of people who were congenial—their intellectual interests and outlooks and so on—a remarkable generosity of spirit in the sense of giving and caring. If someone was in trouble, there was a very gentle way of moving in to support them. People really cared a great deal about each other. . . . There was a great deal of formality, but that kind of formality, I would say, [was] a protection against over-stepping and invading privacy.[43]

There were times when Jack Frost lost his temper and squabbled with his wife. Often as not, the cause was some expense Susan had incurred at a time when the family finances seemed tight to him. "Family finances were quite an issue," recalled their daughter years later. In control even when angry, he rarely shouted, but he raised his voice. "Great Jerusalem!"

Frost would cry and retreat to his study. And Susan would storm off to her room and slam the door. At other times, when preoccupied with some academic matter, Frost would pace up and down the hall and in and out of the dining room "clacking" his teeth. "Jack," his wife would plead angrily, "would you please stop clacking your teeth. It gets on my nerves."[44]

Frost had other mannerisms, and they also occasionally irritated his wife. He talked to himself, sometimes when working on a lecture or paper, sometimes when musing about a nonacademic subject of interest to him, or sometimes as an idle habit. He often held a pencil or other object in his hand, and kept it constantly in motion—jiggling it. And, he was a chain smoker of cigarettes. He worked late into the night when preparing a class or reviewing data, but he was an early—and often grumpy—riser. Up and in the kitchen by 6:30, he was particular about his coffee, preferring the Lady Graham brand. Along with his morning coffee, he read the newspaper, and only after that was he ready to take on the day's work. A tall, thin, almost angular man, he ate sparingly. Kidney stew—one of Eva Anderson's specialties—was a favorite dish.

Frost frequently worked at home, sometimes preparing lectures or problems for his classes, sometimes reviewing the work of his students or colleagues. Especially during the years he served as dean, he often found it useful to bring a coworker to his home in order to work together without the interruptions that administrative duties so often brought. However, at five o'clock in the afternoon, work was put away and Eva Anderson brought out the martini pitcher. Frost liked martinis and was particular in this taste. He always personally mixed the martinis he served.

Frost developed an increasingly close and affectionate relationship with his daughter, whom he called Susie, as she matured. He wrote to her when his work took him away from Baltimore and when she was at school in Winchester, Virginia, or working in Boston. A letter from Cincinnati, which he visited from time to time in his continuing position as director of the field station there, written about 1920, says, "your Daddy has been very bad not to have written sooner," and charges the young girl with taking good care of the family cat Millie's kittens, "just like you were their mummy." In the same letter, Frost also described his plans to visit the Indian mounds in nearby Newark.[45] A decade later, letters apparently written to his daughter away at school are full of family news. On the other hand, the two Susans, mother and daughter, had a sometimes tempestuous relationship. As the daughter matured, she challenged her mother's authority and the resulting friction sometimes generated sparks. "My mother and I did not get on too well. She was just too strong a parent," daughter Susan recalled in 1975.[46] Interestingly, the daughter conscientiously saved all of the letters written to her by her father, but apparently kept none of those from her mother, although it is clear from references in the father's letters that her mother was also writing to her.

As was true for many American families at the time, Sunday afternoon automobile rides were a not infrequent form of weekend diversion and relaxation. The homes of friends and relatives were the usual destinations of Sunday drives. Vaucluse, the Pikesville, Maryland, home of some of Susan Frost's Barton relatives, was a frequent stopping place. So also was Exning in Middleburg, sometimes for a weekend visit, sometimes for just the day. Exning, Susan's childhood home, was now owned by her sister Anne and her husband Thomas Dudley; they had acquired it in the early 1920s after the death of the Haxall parents. Tom Dudley and Jack Frost had become good friends, and they enjoyed sitting and carrying on long dialogues on the large veranda while their wives chatted on the lawn. The three Haxall sisters had a family reputation for their love of talking, and conversations among them often went on for hours. In an August 14, 1933, letter to his daughter in Boston, Frost recounted driving to Exning on Sunday, where he apparently left Susan with her Haxall relatives. He then drove home via Marshall where he visited his sister, Mattie.[47]

Another favorite destination in Middleburg was Glen Ora, the home of Susan's cousins, the Tabb family. One such visit during her childhood was recalled by Susan Frost Parrish as involving a drive down a secondary road so muddy that her father had to put chains on his old Hupmobile to get us through the rutted, slippery mud. . . . Once arrived, [we] found a casual, gentle family who seemed devoted to my parents. Cousin Nell [Tabb] was the type who, when I complained of my shoes hurting, told my mother to let me take them off and go barefoot. . . . A very big dog of theirs, whose tail came level with the surface of the dining room table, . . . swished it and knocked off the teacups.[48]

For the most part, Jack Frost and his family had a rewarding and happy life in Baltimore. Both warmth and humor were present in their home. They were a close and loving family with many friends. They struggled through the Depression, but survived with grace and enjoyed a relatively "upper class" life. They joined clubs that seemed important to them. They sent their daughter to a boarding school in Winchester, Virginia, and gave her a "coming-out party." Daughter Susan was invited to attend the St. Cecilia debutante ball in Charleston, South Carolina, but she declined this social honor.[49] The community of the Johns Hopkins School of Hygiene and Public Health faculty was their community in large measure, but they also maintained close ties with many of Susan's relatives, both in Baltimore and at Exning.

9

Professor

> The most important preparation in epidemiology
> is not any particular amount and kind of
> knowledge but the desire, the determination and
> ability to add to it, for epidemiology is
> concerned not only with the application of
> existing knowledge but more particularly with its
> refinement and extension.
>
> —*Wade Hampton Frost*[1]

The challenges—the tasks and the opportunities—facing Wade Hampton Frost as he took up his post at Johns Hopkins were enormous. He was charged with creating an academic curriculum in a discipline where none existed; indeed, the science of epidemiology was only minimally defined. "Epidemiology" means, literally, the study of that which is upon the people. The word in its Spanish form, *epidemiología*, may have first been used early in the nineteenth century by Joachin de Villalba in writing about diphtheria in Spain. As Frost knew it, the discipline was one of observation and investigation of disease outbreaks, whether by John Snow in his study of cholera in mid-nineteenth-century London or by the Public Health Service team in its efforts to stem an epidemic of yellow fever in New Orleans in 1906. Frost, himself, had investigated outbreaks of typhoid fever, polio, and influenza. Later, epidemiologists would develop statistical techniques and mathematical models that made possible new understanding of the ways in which diseases are transmitted among people, and Frost would contribute in large measure to these advances in methodology and knowledge. But those developments were, as yet, years away.

Much later, with nearly two decades of experience in his academic role behind him, Frost wrote:

> Epidemiology . . . is something more than the total of its established facts. It includes their orderly arrangement into chains of inference which extend . . . beyond the bounds of direct observation.[2]

That elegant and astute perception of his field took time to evolve, both in Frost's wisdom and in the understanding of the field by the communities of working health professionals, scholars of disease, and the interested public.

In the fall of 1919, as Frost faced the immediate challenge of creating a curriculum and a department in epidemiology, he had a greater task than that confronted by today's professors of epidemiology. He could not simply pull together the traditional material covered in such a course and in standard texts, as those trail blazes did not exist. The discipline was present in Europe as a newly emergent, germinating seedling with its roots planted in the nineteenth-century German hygienic institutes of Max von Pettenkofer and Robert Koch. Bacteriologic investigations dominated those institutions, but the idea had emerged that there was something more than the study of microbes to this field of endeavor. In 1928 Frost noted an 1883 definition of epidemiology by August Hirsch who called it "a science which [gives] a picture of the occurrence, the distribution and types of the . . . diseases of mankind."[3]

In Frost's time, epidemiology was being taught in courses in several British universities. Arthur Newsholme, who would become Frost's friend, had studied trends in tuberculosis mortality in Great Britain. There were few American precedents, however, for Frost was the first professor of epidemiology in the first department of epidemiology in the first school of public health in North America. His friends and colleagues, William Sedgwick at the Massachusetts Institute of Technology, and Milton Rosenau, who had left the Hygienic Laboratory for a Harvard University professorship, were giving lectures in sanitary engineering and epidemiology. Victor C. Vaughan was teaching public health at the University of Michigan. Hermann Biggs and Mitchell Pruden were lecturing on public health measures and emphasizing disease surveillance and quarantine in New York City. A department of epidemiology and an entire curriculum in epidemiology were without precedent, however, and Frost faced the challenge of organizing them and deciding what to include and how to present it. There were no texts upon which he could draw.

Frost had received his mandate from William Welch, who (as we saw in chapter 8) more than any other individual had been responsible for the founding of the Johns Hopkins School of Hygiene and Public Health and had obtained funding for the new venture from the Rockefeller Foundation. But the mandate was not sharply defined by Welch, for he operated by making his faculty appointments with great care and then giving his chosen men free rein to pursue the course set for them. Yet it was clear to Welch and to the faculty he recruited to the Johns Hopkins University that the new School of Hygiene and Public Health would do more than simply train sanitarians. The Johns Hopkins faculty, including Frost, would train professionals and leaders of the discipline. More than that, the faculty and their students would advance knowledge in the field by whatever research techniques were appropriate to the task. Frost's mandate was broad in scope.

A scant two months after assuming his new position, Frost was asked to submit a proposal for the organization and development of the new department. His proposal, he wrote, could not be "anything more than tentative" because:

1. The work of organizing this department has just been begun.
2. The field of epidemiology . . . is not yet clearly defined.
3. The field as provisionally defined has not been covered in a systematic manner, so that the scope and methods of instruction must likewise be worked out gradually.[4]

Echoing his disciplinary forbears, few as they were, Frost continued by defining "the special field of epidemiology [as] the natural history of infectious diseases, with special reference to the circumstances which determine their occurrence in nature."[5] He then outlined in careful detail a plan of instruction that would include (1) twenty to thirty lectures covering the principles and methods of the field with illustrative examples; (2) laboratory exercises based on analysis of records of actual epidemiological studies and including the use of statistical analysis of the data in those records; (3) field work by each student; (4) a series of conferences focused on critical review of selected epidemiological studies; and (5) "the development by each student of an assigned topic in epidemiology."[6] The last of these items clearly envisioned a thesis by each student who would come under the principal guidance of his department and its faculty.

Frost then addressed his attention to the role of research in his new department, and noted that it would necessarily be developed cooperatively with a number of agencies. These agencies would include, in his estimation, the United States Public Health Service, of which he was still an officer on active duty, and also the health departments of both Baltimore and the State of Maryland. Additionally, he anticipated collaboration with other departments in the School of Hygiene and Public Health and in the School of Medicine.

Frost concluded his analysis by requesting the appointment of one associate and two instructors, two statistical clerks, and one secretary-stenographer. He felt that this staff would have to be increased in future years. In fact, the staff rarely grew beyond that level. Salaries in the new school were expected to be comparable with those in the preclinical departments of the School of Medicine. Professors were to be paid $5,000 to $6,000 per year, associate professors $2,800 to $3,500, associates $1,800 to $2,500, and instructors and assistants $1,200 to $1,650.[7] Frost asked for salaries at the high end of these ranges. The department occupied three rooms in McCoy Hall on Monument Street at that time, and Frost deemed that space sufficient for the coming year. Figure 9.1 depicts Frost at his desk early in his tenure at Johns Hopkins.

During its early, formative years, the School of Hygiene and Public Health operated with an academic calendar consisting of six "trimesters," each approximately two months in length; later this system evolved into a more traditional quarter system. Into this structure, Frost fit his tripartite program. He planned,

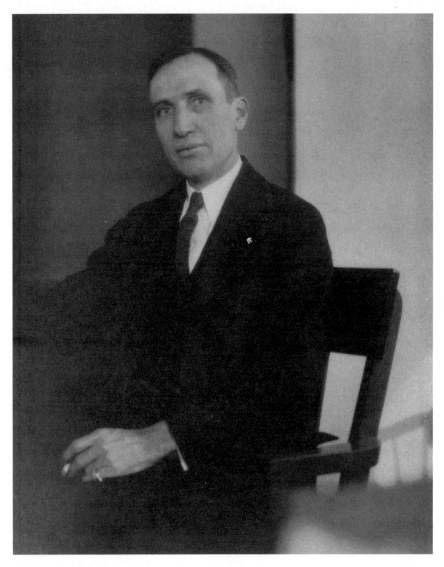

Figure 9.1. Wade Hampton Frost seated at his desk in his office at Johns Hopkins School of Hygiene and Public Health. This photograph was probably taken during the mid 1920s. Photograph is from the Claude Moore Health Sciences Library, University of Virginia Health Sciences Center, Charlottesville, VA: Wade Hampton Frost Archives, Box 6, Folder 53. Reproduced with permission, courtesy of the Historical Collection and Services of the Claude Moore Health Sciences Library.

developed, and taught a series of lectures. He added to them laboratories focusing on actual epidemic situations. Finally, each student was required to work on a problem, and Frost or another professor served as mentor, preceptor, and critic for the student in this effort. As in the academic world today, research at Johns Hopkins under the leadership of William Welch and William H. Howell was expected of every professor. Frost had already demonstrated his capacity to contribute new knowledge in his investigations of water contamination, of poliomyelitis, and of influenza. In each of these areas he had made and understood observations that advanced medical knowledge. As Frost developed problems for his epidemiology students, he put the neophyte students into the research arena, and under his guiding hand they joined him in contributing to research in the field as they dealt with the problems assigned to them.

Initially, three courses in epidemiology were offered: Epidemiology 1, Epidemiology 2, and Epidemiology 3.[8] Epidemiology 1, which was offered for the first time in the spring of 1920, met for three half day-long sessions each week—one hour of lecture followed by a three hour laboratory exercise. In subsequent years Epidemiology 1 was followed by Epidemiology 2, which also required a basic knowledge of statistics as a prerequisite. Epidemiology 2 covered the same material as Epidemiology 1, but more critically and in greater detail. Epidemiology 3 was made up of special studies—the student field work leading to a thesis. As Frost's tenure in the department continued, a small number of additional courses were added. A series of special lectures was arranged as a course. Field trips were added. And, notably, a joint course in epidemiology and biostatistics developed and taught by Frost and Lowell Reed became a linchpin in the training of Johns Hopkins epidemiology students. In fact, this course soon assumed the position of Epidemiology 2 and was required of every student.

One of Frost's first challenges at Johns Hopkins was to recruit a faculty to teach the students who would soon be enrolled.

In this he appears to have been helped by his friends and former colleagues, William Sedgwick and Milton Rosenau, then both in Boston and teaching public health in a joint program of the Massachusetts Institute of Technology and Harvard. Frost made his initial faculty appointments in 1921. W. Thurber Fales had received a Doctor of Science degree from Harvard the previous year, a graduate of the Sedgwick-Rosenau program. Fales remained on the Johns Hopkins faculty for three years before moving to the Alabama State Board of health as the director of its bureau of vital statistics. Milton V. Veldee also joined Frost's faculty in 1921, staying on for only one academic year. Veldee had served as a bacteriologist with Frost in Cincinnati. He then studied medicine and received a Doctor of Medicine degree from Harvard in 1919 and may also have been recommended by Rosenau or Sedgwick. He left Johns Hopkins after only one year to join the Public Health Service.

In 1922 Frost was joined by James A. Doull. Doull was one of Frost's closest and most trusted associates, and they became good friends. Doull was originally appointed as an associate and named the school's first associate professor in 1926. He was a Canadian physician who had studied public health at Cambridge University in England. Thereafter, he attended the Johns Hopkins School of Hygiene and Public Health where he received his doctorate in 1921. He was then asked to join the faculty. In fact, many of the early faculty members were graduates of the school; there were at that time few other venues for academic training in public health. Doull remained at Johns Hopkins until 1930, when he moved to Cleveland to become professor of hygiene and public health at Western Reserve University (now Case Western Reserve University) School of Medicine.

George Ramsey was Frost's fourth faculty appointment. He joined the department in 1926 as an associate, being promoted to associate professor in 1930 to take the slot vacated by Doull. A native of the Allegheny Mountain city of Olean, New York, he attended Rutgers University and then received his M.D. degree from Columbia University in 1917. After serving in the army in World War I, he was a resident physician at the Herman

Kiefer Hospital, a tuberculosis hospital in Detroit, from 1919 to 1920. In 1920 he joined the Michigan Department of Health, and the following year became Deputy Commissioner of Health for Michigan. He was a student at the School of Hygiene and Public Health in 1923 and 1924. Ramsey left Johns Hopkins in 1933 to join the New York State Health Department and became Assistant Commissioner of Preventable Diseases. He later served as Health Commissioner for Westchester County, New York.

Miriam Brailey became the department's first female faculty member in 1932, one year after she received the Doctor of Public Health degree from the school. Initially an instructor, she was promoted to associate in 1936. A pediatrician, Brailey's doctoral thesis was based on a study of tuberculosis in children seen at the Harriet Lane Home, Johns Hopkins Hospital's pediatric unit. As a faculty member, she remained active in the study of pediatric tuberculosis in Baltimore. She served as the director of the Harriet Lane Tuberculosis Clinic, and in 1941 she became head of the Bureau of Tuberculosis of the Baltimore City Health Department.

Table 9.1 lists the faculty members of the Johns Hopkins Department of Epidemiology during Frost's tenure as its chairman. Many of the appointees served for only a few years. Many were recent graduates of Frost's program. For the most part, Frost had only two or three individuals working with him; his was never the large academic empire that many such departments—including the present one at Johns Hopkins— became in later years as the discipline expanded.

Although William Welch clearly intended that the new School of Hygiene and Public Health would serve as a research institute and would train physicians in the academic disciplines of public health, the school's founder also recognized that it would have to teach aspects of public health that he considered somewhat mundane. Thus it was that he established a Department of Public Health Administration. To teach this subject, Welch recruited Sir Arthur Newsholme, who had recently retired from a distinguished career in public health in England. He had served as Chief Medical Officer for the Local Government Board

Table 9.1.
Faculty of the Department of Epidemiology of the Johns Hopkins School of Hygiene and Public Health during the tenure of Wade Hampton Frost, 1919–1938.

Years	Name	Rank
1919–1938	Wade Hampton Frost	Resident Lecturer (1919–1921); Professor (1921–1938)
1921–1922	Milton V. Veldee	Instructor
1921–1924	W. Thurber Fales	Instructor
1922–1930	James A. Doull	Associate (1922–1926); Associate Professor (1926–1930)
1926–1933	George H. Ramsey	Associate (1926–1930); Associate Professor (1930–1933)
1930–1936	Vivian Van Volkenburgh	Associate
1930–1931	Howard C. Stewart	Associate
1930–1931	Edwin L. McQuade	Instructor
1930–1931	James A. Crabtree	Associate
1932–1959	Miriam E. Brailey	Instructor (1932–1936); Associate (1936–1959)
1933–1935	Alexander G. Gilliam	Instructor
1935–1936	Floyd M. Feldmann	Instructor
1936–1937	Howard C. Stewart	Associate
1937–1946	John J. Phair	Associate (1937–1943); Associate Professor (1943–1946)
1937–	Perrin H. Long	Lecturer

of Great Britain, a position somewhat akin to that of Surgeon General of the Public Health Service in the United States. He was a strong advocate of socialized medicine and a national health service. Newsholme spent two years in Baltimore as a resident lecturer, and when he departed, Frost was given the task of teaching public health administration. Frost brought Newsholme, with whom he had become a close friend, back to Baltimore as guest lecturer from time to time, but beginning in 1922 Frost served as chairman of the Department of Public Health Administration and carried much of the burden of teaching this subject. Frost tried unsuccessfully to entice Hermann Biggs to take over the department. He then recruited Allen Weir Freeman to this post. Freeman, then a Public Health Service officer, had worked with Frost in the study of the 1916 New York City polio epidemic. Subsequently he had served as Health

Commissioner for Ohio and reorganized the health department of that state. With Freeman at the helm, Frost relinquished his role in the Department of Public Health Administration. Freeman spent the remainder of his career at the Johns Hopkins School of Hygiene and Public Health; he was elected dean of the faculty for a three year term in 1934, following Frost in that post.

In 1921 Frost was promoted to professor. His salary was $3,000 per year.[9] Since he was still a commissioned officer of the Public Health Service, this amount was probably in addition to his service pay. Despite his success at the School of Hygiene and Public Health, Frost found the task of serving two masters—Johns Hopkins University and the United States Public Health Service—difficult at times. As early as March 14, 1921, he wrote to Surgeon General Hugh Cumming noting that his Public Health Service orders "appear simply to lend my services to the School without any compensating advantage to the Service." He suggested a luncheon meeting to discuss the issue, which apparently did not take place.[10]

In the summer of 1922 Cumming wrote to Frost telling him that he was contemplating establishing a Division of Scientific Research within the Public Health Service and asking Frost if he would be interested in assuming the post of its director.[11] Frost replied promptly, tactfully expressing his willingness to be assigned wherever he could best serve but making it clear that he was not really interested in the position.[12] Frost had ambivalent feelings about his dual masters. Although he indicated that did not want to leave Johns Hopkins, he told Cumming that he had "never felt inclined to consider really seriously" resigning from the Public Health Service. "What I really want to do . . . is get the work on stream pollution more firmly on its feet."[13]

Time passed, and on January 3, 1926 he penned a personal note to William Welch, which he passed first to William Howell for review before sending it on to Welch.

> I am sure you know that, consulting my personal wishes and comfort, I would unhesitatingly prefer to stay at the school; but I am by no

means certain that I can be as useful in the School as in the Service. After more than twenty years in the Service I feel that I know its "machinery" pretty well and know how to use it as a working tool.[14]

Welch's reply has not been preserved. However, a hand-written note from Surgeon General Hugh Cumming dated June 20, 1929, expresses "personal as well as official regret" at having just signed the acceptance of Frost's resignation of his commission. "My regret," he wrote, "is not so much the loss of your technical and professional ability as the loss of you as a gentleman whose ideas and actions have been an inspiration to the other officers who have been thrown with you."[15] Frost's resignation took effect on August 8, 1929. He would now be a full-time academician, although his national stature was such that his arena was not limited to his home base in Baltimore.

His career path now irrevocably set in academia, Frost turned to teaching and training those who would follow the trail of his footprints. He worked hard at preparing his lectures, writing them out before each class, frequently completely in narrative fashion, sometimes as detailed outlines. He built his presentations around case studies—epidemics and outbreaks—that were classics in epidemiological investigation or were those in which he had been personally involved. He was interested in the formal discipline of logic, and he used its techniques to develop the points he wished to make in his presentations. When it came time for him to deliver his carefully prepared expositions, Frost did not read them; he had committed to memory their contents, if not their words, in the process of their preparation.

His enormous efforts at preparation did not make Frost a good lecturer, however. In the lecture hall he stood at the blackboard, pencil or more often chalk in constant motion in one hand, cigarette in the other. As he talked, he often faced the blackboard, talking to the blackboard, as it were, and making it difficult for those in the back of the room to hear him. He did not write more than an occasional word or brief phrase with the chalk he held. Rather, he tapped the board with the chalk making a series of dots when he wanted to emphasize a point. He took his glasses off and replaced them frequently as he talked. From time to time he stopped to puff on his cigarette. His choice of words was elegant; he had a marvelous command of the English language and an aptitude for choosing the right word and the best phrase to express his meaning. Yet, his tone of speech was monotonous. Figure 9.2 depicts Frost in the lecture hall, standing at the black board with chalk in hand, notes, slide rule, and reference books on the table in front of him.

Some of his students later described Frost's lectures as elegant and comprehensive; some of them called them boring. They were detailed and complete with much substance. Yet, "about half the students . . . went to sleep."[16] "He was not . . . a good Danny Kaye, [but he] was tremendous in substance."[17] Ernest Stebbins, who took Frost's lecture course in epidemiology in 1929 and who would later himself become dean of the Johns Hopkins School of Hygiene and Public Health, reflected as follows:

> [It was said] a number of times that Frost was such a dull lecturer. I just couldn't understand it because, no, he wasn't flamboyant, he didn't make you laugh, he didn't shower you with oratory, but he made everything just so clear and concise, and you could just see that he had worked over these lectures repeatedly and had spotted where it would be difficult for a student that wasn't familiar with epidemiology to get confused, and he repeated—some people object to that—but he did it in order to be very sure that his point was clear.[18]

Morton Levin recalled Frost's lectures:

> He did not have a forceful manner of presentation, but he was always intensely interested in what he was presenting, and sometimes he became so interested that you could see him thinking out loud, so to speak . . . and sometimes forgetting that there was a class listening in.[19]

The effort expended by Frost in preparing his lectures is well illustrated by lectures given on the collection of epidemiological data during the early years of his course in epidemiology.[20] His outline for this lecture in 1920 comprises three typewritten pages with extensive handwritten notes in the margins. The outline itself is sparse in detail. It focuses on demographic

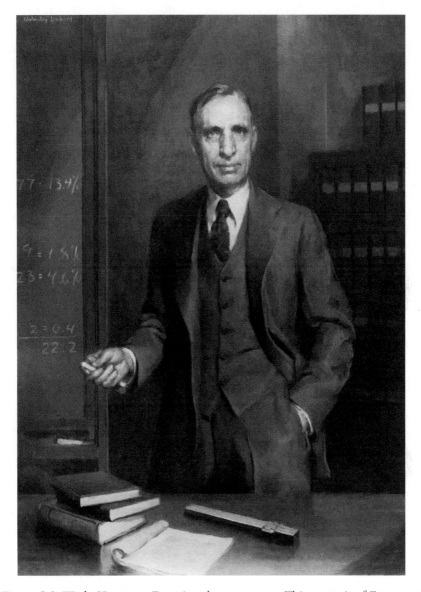

Figure 9.2. Wade Hampton Frost in a lecture room. This portrait of Frost was painted by Walmsley Lenhard in 1939. It now hangs in the Frost Seminar Room of the Department of Epidemiology, Johns Hopkins Bloomberg School of Public Health, Baltimore, Maryland. Photograph is from the Wade Hampton Frost Archives, Claude Moore Health Sciences Library, University of Virginia Health Sciences Center, Charlottesville, Virginia. Reproduced with permission, courtesy of the Historical Collection and Services of the Claude Moore Health Sciences Library.

characteristics of the study population, including reference to such sources of information for the community as census reports, tax books, school records, and sanitary and other surveys that may have been carried out in the community. Clearly Frost was drawing on his own experience in the investigations of epidemics of typhoid fever, polio, and influenza.

The outlines for the following two years are each six typewritten pages long and much more detailed. In 1922, the concepts taught by Frost had evolved far beyond the procedures for data collection to include the need for the "formulation of a working hypothesis, envisiging [*sic*] all the conditions (determinable) which may be supposed to have an influence upon the occurrence of the disease."[21] The types of data that might be collected are listed in Frost's outline in great detail, and tabular data from investigation of a typhoid fever outbreak in Little Rock, Arkansas, are included. Pencilled marginal notes in Frost's handwriting make reference to studies of pellagra and influenza as well as shell fish-related disease. Representative of the detail Frost characteristically proposed for investigations is a pencilled note suggesting contacting the local plumbers union for information. If Frost put great effort into his teaching effort, it must also be said that he anticipated that those whom he taught would expend great effort in their public health careers. Frost himself had become a compulsive collector and obsessive organizer of epidemiological data, and he clearly expected his students to develop similar habits.

Most of Frost's lectures dealt with individual diseases and explored in great depth their epidemiologies. Frost presented great classic epidemiologic studies of certain diseases. Both Snow's work on cholera and Budd's on typhoid were presented to the students, who were encouraged to read the original papers, for which Frost provided the references. Frost felt that these studies as reported originally were, in his words, "apt to be unusually clear and instructive" and that "much of this quality is lost in second-hand accounts." He urged his friend William Welch to use his influence to have the Institute of Medical History at Johns Hopkins republish some of these great works.[22]

It is notable that Snow's studies of cholera, considered models of epidemiological investigation by Frost and now repeatedly cited as classic studies, were by and large ignored in Snow's time and for the ensuing seventy-five years. Robert Koch, who identified the organism that causes cholera in 1884, seems to have been unaware of Snow's work. In fact, it was Frost who brought Snow's work forth to the medical public.[23] At Frost's instigation, two of Snow's seminal papers were reprinted in 1936 by the Commonwealth Fund with an introduction by Frost.[24]

Frost presented the work of Peter Ludwig Panum to his students in one of his lectures. Panum was a young Danish medical officer who was sent to the Faroe Islands in 1846 to provide medical care to the victims of a measles epidemic then raging there. Measles had not been present on these isolated islands for sixty-five years when it was reintroduced. Panum's careful inquiries and observations established for the first time (1) that the incubation period was thirteen to fourteen days prior to the development of the rash, (2) that measles was always infectious in origin and transmitted person-to-person and not by fomites in the environments previously frequented by patients, and (3) that immunity to measles was life-long. These early observations of Panum clearly fit into the mold of Frost's "chains of inference which extend . . . beyond the bounds of direct observation."[25] In 1924 Frost commissioned a translation of Panum's Danish monograph by Ada Sommerville Hatcher of the Public Health Service for his use in teaching; this translation was later published by the Delta Omega Society, a national honor society for students of public health founded at Johns Hopkins in 1924.[26] How Frost came to be aware of Panum's work, which had previously been published only in Danish in 1885, is not known; one can surmise that his friend Arthur Newsholme might have told him of it.

In other lectures Frost drew upon his own experiences and those of his colleagues with polio, typhoid, diphtheria, and influenza. For example, Frost presented a two-part lecture on typhoid in his Epidemiology 1 course describing an epidemic of typhoid in Decatur and New Decatur, Alabama. The outbreak occurred in the winter of 1914–1915 and was investigated by Paul Preble, a Public Health Service officer who had been stationed at the time in Cincinnati with Frost. Frost's lecture outline is enormously detailed.[27] It includes census data, maps, records of cases including both demographic and clinical information, and bacteriologic data on various water supply and sewage disposal systems. Frost charted the time course of the outbreak. He discussed the ways in which the raw data should be processed, organized, and analyzed. He summarized what he considered to be notable facts of this epidemic and developed hypotheses concerning the outbreak that could be tested against the data.

Laboratory exercises were an integral part of Frost's curriculum. They followed each of his lectures and were generally closely related to the subject of the lecture. Students were given raw data from epidemiological investigations and expected to analyze them. For these exercises, they were provided with slide rules, which they were expected to return at the end of the course, and sets of reprints, also to be returned; electronic calculators, computers, and copying machines were yet to be invented. Students were expected to equip themselves with graph paper, pen, and ruler.

Reflecting on these laboratory exercises, Ernest Stebbins recalled:

> That was where he really was able to get to the student. Everybody just felt that that was the most wonderful experience. . . . We always worked in groups of about four, five, or six at a table, and we were given these problems, the bare data, and even in the beginning he would have you go through and tabulate directly from the histories, the individual histories, so that you had to go through the whole process. And then you were given questions to answer and suggestions. Not in the beginning; you had to ask how do you go about dealing with a set of figures of this kind. And then he would circulate around . . . and he would ask very probing questions—why did you feel that that was the most suspect source of infection—things of that kind. But he never left the table without giving you some hints as to what you might experiment with. He wouldn't tell you what to do, but he would give you hints.[28]

Similarly, Morton Levin recalled Frost as a probing, questioning teacher, both in laboratory exercises and in the lecture hall.

> There was something about the way Dr. Frost approached both formal teaching and the kind of teaching that went on when you were doing a problem or a thesis which was extremely stimulating because you could see that he was questioning at every point. At every step of the way he was questioning his own premises, as well as yours, as well as any conclusion that you reached. He took nothing for granted, and . . . he took great delight in pointing out inconsistencies, and what he used to call "jokers," the things which seemed to be one way and actually were not, or were explainable by something unforeseen.[29]

As in his lectures, Frost used real cases, often from his own experience, for his laboratory exercises. For example, Exercise 6 of the Epidemiology 1 course given in 1927 was based on his investigation of the bacteriology of the water supply of Washington, D.C., conducted while he was stationed at the Hygienic Laboratory. The directions for this exercise comprised six single spaced, typewritten pages.[30] They directed students to read Frost's sixty-nine page paper on the subject published in 1911.[31] Demographic data and population maps were to be extracted from the published paper. Frost also provided detailed data on the occurrence of typhoid in Washington from 1906 to 1909. Students were then posed a series of questions designed to establish the relationship of typhoid to water supply, milk supply, and the use of privies. Similarly, Exercise 7 was based on Frost's investigation of the 1916 polio outbreak in the New York City area; it made use of both the published report and detailed data provided to the students in tabular form.

When Abel Wolman, a sanitary engineer at the University of Maryland, accepted an appointment at Johns Hopkins in 1937, he made it a condition of his appointment that he could send his Maryland sanitary engineering students to Johns Hopkins to take courses in epidemiology, biometry (biomedical statistics; a term invented at Johns Hopkins, probably by Raymond Pearl, perhaps by Lowell Reed), and physiology taught at Johns Hopkins by Frost and his faculty colleagues. More than that, Wolman wanted his engineering students paired with the mostly physician public health students. Frost was skeptical, but agreed, only to find that the engineering students excelled, outpacing the physicians, because the engineers were "mathematically inclined." They had the habits of precise, mathematical, logical thinking that Frost had acquired and brought to the medical field of epidemiology.[32]

Frost expected his students not only to learn what he had taught but also to be able to think and reason in the arena of epidemiology. On March 11, 1927, he gave a four-hour examination at the conclusion of the Epidemiology 1 course.[33] Five questions were listed, with students expected to answer four of them. The questions were probing. The first two asked students to detail the data needed and methods of collecting it for epidemics of typhoid and scarlet fever. The third and fourth asked students to discuss the natural history of polio and influenza and explain the occurrence of outbreaks of these diseases. The final question asked students to plan an investigation of the relationship between childhood tuberculosis and malnutrition. With an hour for each of the four chosen questions, students were given ample opportunity to demonstrate their mastery of the concepts Frost and his colleagues had taught.

We have seen that Frost had many friends and collaborators among his faculty colleagues. None of these friendships was more notable than that with Lowell Reed of the department of biometry and biostatistics. Margaret Merrell relates that the two men first met while Frost was pacing the corridor "shaking colored balls from one box to another to explore chance effects in the progress of an epidemic."[34] In fact, Frost often paced the corridors when his mind was wrestling with a problem. He enjoyed the mathematical aspects of his discipline. Such an epidemiologist would surely be attractive to the statistician-mathematician, Reed. Soon the two men were teaching together. Their course, which was first taught in 1925, was jointly offered as Epidemiology 2 and Biostatistics 9. Like Frost, Reed believed that the most effective teaching mode was that of small group exercises. The 1934 schedule for this course listed twenty-two lectures and five laboratory exercises, most of the latter stretching over several days. Epidemic theory and statistical methods, largely taught by Reed, were intermingled with examples drawn from the epidemiology of influenza, common colds, and tuberculosis, taught by Frost.[35]

The collaboration with Lowell Reed did more than provide a stimulating course for Johns Hopkins students. It generated new ideas in the minds of the two men, and from these ideas some important contributions to epidemiological methodology. Life table methods were first developed during the 1820s and 1830s, perhaps first by William Farr, a statistician appointed in the Registrar-General's Office of Great Britain in 1838. They had been in use for some time in the insurance industry. These methods permit the adjustment of population sizes at intervals so that accurate year-to-year risks related to observed disease effects can be assessed. Drawing on his experience in teaching this course, Frost used this technique, which he and Reed further refined, to study mortality from tuberculosis.

One of the most significant scientific products of the Frost-Reed collaboration was the first mathematical expression of what is called the epidemic curve, which is sometimes known as the Reed-Frost model of epidemics. At the heart of this concept is the understanding that each infectious case can infect a number of susceptible individuals in a population. As more individuals are infected, develop disease, and subsequently become immune to reinfection, the number of individuals that can be infected decreases. Ultimately, with a falling number of susceptible persons in the population, the epidemic must wane. Two three-page outlines, one dated March 8, 1927, the other undated, carefully develop this concept.[36] Frost drafted, but never published, a full scientific paper describing the concept in detail. Reed also began a draft manuscript, but it was destroyed by a fire in his house, and he did not resume the project. In 1976, when Philip E. Sartwell was editor of the *American Journal of Epidemiology*, he published Frost's paper with a figure drawn by him from Frost's tabular data.[37] (This figure is reproduced as figure 9.3.) In 1967, Floyd Feldmann, one of Frost's former students and junior faculty members who was

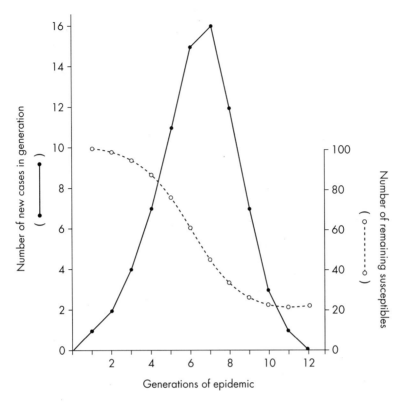

Figure 9.3. Epidemic curve derived from Frost's data, starting with one case added to a population of 100 susceptibles, and assuming that each individual has contact with two others during the infectious period of the disease; and number of remaining susceptibles at each time period. Frost WH. Some concepts of epidemics in general. *Am J Epidemiology.* 1976; 103:141–51. Reproduced with permission.

then at Cornell University, joined with colleagues to publish one of the first attempts to model the epidemiology of tuberculosis using Frost's and Reed's concepts.[38] Feldmann's 1935 Johns Hopkins doctoral thesis had been based on an investigation of tuberculosis in Baltimore under Frost's guidance.

Why neither Frost nor Reed published any of the methodological advances they developed during their joint teaching remains a curious enigma. Frost did contribute a review of epidemiology to a 1928 medical text—his only publication dealing substantially with epidemiological methods—but this chapter is fairly general in nature and lacks detail. He did point out in this work that highly infectious diseases producing a high degree of immunity, including measles and yellow fever, "would die out in any but a large population." On the other hand, "with low immunizing properties, . . . the result would be almost universal *recurrent* attacks."[39] But beyond this text chapter, nothing appeared in print, although the work of many students firmly established the techniques of Frost and Reed in the methodology of epidemiology.

Since field experience for each student was an expectation of the founders of the new school, it was soon apparent that appropriate sites for these experiences would have to be developed. Both an urban and a more rural center for teaching and demonstration were sought. The first of these to be established was the Washington County Training Center in Hagerstown, Maryland. In 1911, the newly created Hagerstown Civic League, whose members included many of the leading women of the community, joined with the Maryland Association for the Prevention and Relief of Tuberculosis to raise money to support a public health nurse in the county health department. This community effort attracted the attention of the leaders of the School of Hygiene and Public Health, and in 1921 the Washington County Health Demonstration was established with support from the Maryland State Health Department, The United States Public Health Service, the Rockefeller Foundation, and the Security Cement and Lime Company of Hagerstown. While this unit provided significant measures of service to the Hagerstown community and while it served as a major research base for a number of Public Health Service studies, it was not successful as a training site for Johns Hopkins public health students. It was too far from Baltimore—six hours by the transportation modes of the early 1920s—to make access easy for students. Moreover, in order not to disturb the didactic curriculum, students were sent to the center for periods of only one week, a time too short to allow involvement in any on-going studies. Finally, the Johns Hopkins faculty rarely visited the center.[40]

If the Washington County unit in Hagerstown did not serve the school and its students well, the opposite was true for the urban center developed largely under the leadership of Frost. The Eastern Health District of Baltimore encompassed roughly one square mile adjacent to the Johns Hopkins medical institutions.[41] It was a neighborhood of row houses, and many of its approximately sixty thousand inhabitants were recent immigrants. During the 1920s a number of attempts were made by members of the Johns Hopkins medical and nursing faculties to use this district for educational and research activities, but they were largely rebuffed by the health professionals practicing in the area. In 1930, Huntington Williams, a graduate of the Johns Hopkins School of Hygiene and Public Health, became Baltimore's health commissioner and Harry Mustard commissioner for the district, and with that a new era of cooperation dawned. Frost used his contacts to secure funding from both the Rockefeller Foundation and the Public Health Service.

The purposes of the Eastern Health District program were enunciated in a School of Hygiene and Public Health draft prepared in March 1932. They were:

1. To furnish facilities for the field training of workers now employed or to be employed by the agencies conducting public health activities in the city, and of the students of public health enrolled in the teaching institution.
2. To furnish a field for more precise and instructive study of numerous public health problems, both administrative and epidemiological.[42]

It should be noted that this statement begins with the objective on improving the training of *"workers now employed or to be employed by the agencies conducting public health activities in the city."* The school's faculty expected not just to train its students and conduct research but also to improve public health work in the district and greater Baltimore.

The good will of the community was secured through the tireless efforts of Williams and Mustard, and a remarkable series of studies began. Many of these, as evidenced by the titles of theses listed in table 9.2, were done under Frost's

Table 9.2.
Students at the Johns Hopkins School of Hygiene
and Public Health for whom Wade Hampton Frost served as
thesis advisor or important mentor.*

Name	Year of degree	Thesis title
Reginald M. Atwater	1921	Epidemiological Studies on Diphtheria, 1920–1921.
James A. Doull	1921	Unknown.
Huntington Williams	1921	Unknown.
Frank Coughlin	1922	Unknown.
Archibald Dean	1923	Unknown.
Eugene L. Bishop	1923	Unknown.
George H. Ramsey	1924	Unknown.
Fred L. Soper	1925	Unknown.
G. Foard McGinnes	1928	An Epidemiological Study of Typhoid Fever as Observed in Baltimore, Maryland, During the Winter Months. 1924–1928.
Vivian A. Van Volkenburgh	1929	A Study of the Respiratory Diseases Prevailing in a Group of Families Residing in Baltimore, Maryland, from October 1928 to March 1929.
James B. Black	1929	A Comparative Study of Susceptibility to Diphtheria in the White and Negro Races.
Yoshio Kusama	1929	A Study of Carrier Infection among the Family Associates of Diphtheria Cases in Baltimore, 1920–1929.
Adrian R. Foley	1931	A Study of Tuberculosis in Gibson County, Tennessee: I. Mortality, 1919–1929; II. Prevalence of Infection.
Howard C. Stewart	1931	The Epidemiology of Tuberculosis in Gibson County, Tennessee; A Study of the Prevalence of Tuberculous Infection in 389 Families.
Miriam E. Brailey	1931	A Preliminary Analysis of Certain Records of the Tuberculosis Clinic of the Harriet Lane Home: I. Tuberculous Infection in Children of Tuberculous Families; II. The History to Adolescence of Children Shown to be Tuberculous during Infancy.
Anil C. Chatterji	1931	A Study of Evidence Bearing on the Immunity Conferred by the Common Cold.
Ayodhya N. Das	1932	A Study of the Trend of Age Selection of Poliomyelitis in the United States since 1910.
James A. Crabtree	1932	A Study of the Prevalence and Mortality of Tuberculosis in the Negro Population of Kingsport, Tennessee.
Ernest L. Stebbins	1932	Unknown.
Ralph E. Wheeler	1932	A Study of Mortality and Morbidity in Children Exposed to Household Contact with Pulmonary Tuberculosis in Adults.
James E. Perkins	1933	A Study of the Cases of Tuberculosis Reported in the Eastern Health District.

Table 9.2. (continued)

Name	Year of degree	Thesis Title
Sterling Smith Cook	1934	Cerebrospinal Fever in the United States Navy, 1901–1930.
Charles Howe Eller	1934	Tuberculous Infection and Mortality of Children Exposed to Household Contact with Pulmonary Tuberculosis.
Alexander G. Gilliam	1934	A Study of the Cases of Tuberculosis Reported in the Eastern Health District during the Years 1923–1932, Inclusive.
Morton Loeb Levin	1934	A Comparison of Certain Factors in the Epidemiology of Diphtheria in Baltimore in 1921–22 and in 1933–34.
Floyd M. Feldmann	1935	Tuberculosis Service in the Eastern Health District; A Review of Procedures and Results of the Investigation and Care of Cases.
Margaret Barnard	1935	Unknown.
Ross L. Gauld	1936	A Study of Reported Cases of Tuberculosis and Their Family Contacts.
James Watt	1936	A Study of Infection and Mortality in Children Exposed to Household Contact with Pulmonary Tuberculosis.
Albert Victor Hardy	1936	The Epidemiology of Bacillary Dysentery (A Preliminary Study).
William T. Clark	1937	Investigation of Cases of Recently Acquired Syphilis in Buffalo.
Robert Dyar	1938	Tuberculosis in the Eastern Health District. An Appraisal of Administrative Procedures Based on a Study of Recently Discharged Cases.
Carl A.W. Barkhaus	1938	Tuberculosis in the Eastern Health District. The Selection of Households Associated with Deaths from Tuberculosis.
John J. Phair	1938	The Selection of Tuberculosis in the Eastern Health District.
Leonard Adolph Dewey	1939	A Study of the Prevalence of Syphilis among the Employees of a Large Institution.

*This table was compiled from a review of doctoral theses in the library of the Department of Epidemiology at the Johns Hopkins Bloomberg School of Public Health and other sources, including notes made by Susan Frost Parrish. It is almost certainly incomplete, especially for the earlier years. A number of thesis titles are unknown, and copies of them are no longer available at Johns Hopkins.

supervision. Acute respiratory infections came under scrutiny by Frost and his students, and as time moved on tuberculosis became the most commonly studied disease.

Frost's interest in the epidemiology of tuberculosis fostered studies of this disease in Baltimore not only in the Eastern

Health District. Under the leadership of Edwards A. Park, Professor of Pediatrics and Pediatrician-in-chief of the Johns Hopkins Hospital, the Harriet Lane Pediatric Tuberculosis Clinic was established. Miriam Brailey, a pediatrician who trained in epidemiology with Frost, wrote her thesis on studies she conducted at this clinic. She then joined his faculty, became the director of the clinic, and carried out important longitudinal studies of tuberculosis in children with Frost's support.

Perhaps the greatest impact of Wade Hampton Frost on the many students who came through the school was a result of his mentoring activities. Each student was required to write a thesis, and Frost and his faculty colleagues reviewed draft after draft of these documents. Students both dreaded and looked forward to Frost's comments on their work. They referred to his meticulous critiques as "Frosting." Rigorous though his criticisms sometimes were, he never antagonized students by his reviews, and most of them loved him especially for these one-on-one critique sessions. Sometimes, especially during the years when Frost served as dean, review sessions with students were held at the Frost home in Roland Park, professor and pupil sitting side-by-side on the porch. Frost delighted in finding inconsistencies, mistakes, or fallacious assumptions. "I used to love having him go over my work," James Perkins recalled, "because he'd say, 'you see the joker in that, don't you?'" "I should have picked it up myself, but I didn't."[43]

It is a truism that a professor can be judged by his or her students, and Frost's students were a remarkable group of individuals who went on to accomplishing careers. A partial list of them is provided in table 9.2. A photograph taken in 1936 of Frost with some of his students is reproduced in figure 9.4. Many of Frost's students spent their careers in state or district health departments. Some found academic positions, often of eminence; it has already been noted that a number of them joined the Johns Hopkins faculty, sometimes later moving on to other positions. Some achieved national prominence. Among those in the latter group, Alexander G. Gilliam became a medical director at the National Institutes of Health; Fred L. Soper became Director of

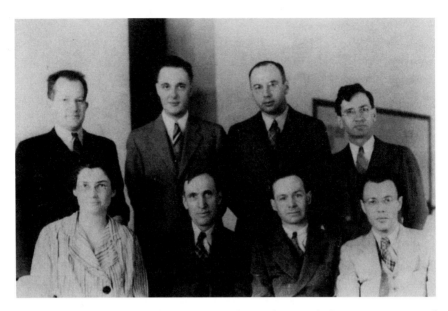

Figure 9.4. Wade Hampton Frost with students of the Department of Epidemiology in 1936. Top row (left to right): Harry Timbres, James Watt, William T. Clark, Albert B. Hardy. Bottom row (left to right): Miriam Brailey, Wade Hampton Frost, Ross Gauld, and Morton Levin. From the archives of the Department of Epidemiology. Johns Hopkins Bloomberg School of Public Health. Reproduced with permission.

the Pan American Sanitary Bureau and oversaw its reorganization as the Pan American Health Organization, the regional office of the World Health Organization for the Americas; G. Foard McGinnes became the National Medical Director of the American Red Cross; and James E. Perkins became Managing Director of the National Tuberculosis Association.

In 1931 the School of Hygiene and Public Health gave up its system of governance by a director, the post in which William Welch and William Howell had served, and began electing deans to three-year terms. Howell had retired, and the university board of trustees accepted a committee recommendation that a dean be elected by department chairs from among their number for a nonrenewable three-year term. Frost was the first faculty member elected to this position by his peers.[44] While he certainly felt honored by this recognition, he also found the duties of the post burdensome nuisances. He continued to teach and to mentor students during these three years, more frequently meeting with his students at his home, often on weekends. As one of his students recalled, "he was more interested in epidemiology than in being dean."[45]

Frost was not only recognized by his students and faculty peers at Johns Hopkins. He also remained active in his discipline and became increasingly nationally prominent in it. He was awarded honors and asked to serve on major advisory boards. He was a prominent member of the American Public Health Association and served on its Governing Council for many years. He served terms as chair of both the Laboratory Section and the Epidemiology Section of the association.

Numerous invitations to travel abroad came to Frost. He turned them down, often passing on the opportunities to James Doull or George Ramsey. He was asked to go to Brazil to develop a course in epidemiology at the Oswaldo Cruz Institute in Rio de Janeiro. His wife and daughter were entranced with the idea, but he could not be persuaded to go. Doull and Allen Freeman went in his place. Evidently the love of travel and adventure of his early Revenue Cutter Service days had passed.

Following his resignation of his Public Health Service commission, Frost remained on the service roster as a consultant in water pollution until his death. His interest in this field continued through many years. He used epidemics of waterborne disease in his teaching, as we have seen. Periodically he revisited and reviewed the activities of the Cincinnati field station, which had reopened after the end of World War I. He attended a number of conferences on water purity held by the Public Health Service or similar agencies. In 1923 he discussed the sources of water pollution in a paper addressed to engineers.[46] In 1924 he and his Cincinnati colleagues assembled a comprehensive review of the findings of the Cincinnati unit with respect to the state of Ohio River water. Frost took the lead in the bacteriologic section of this report.[47] The following year he attended a national meeting of sanitary engineers held in Cincinnati and presented a review of current sewage and drinking water conditions in the United States and of the work of the Public Health Service in this field. He attended the 1925, 1926, and 1927 annual meetings of American state and territorial public health officers held in Washington, D.C., and participated in their discussions of water pollution. In these meetings he also commented on the problems of shell fish and disease vectors, since in 1925 he had been appointed chairman of a Public Health Service committee to make recommendations concerning the sanitary control of oysters. In his comments he displayed a precise knowledge of public health regulations related to the shell fish industry.

Frost's continuing interest in water quality makes it clear that he was not simply an academic epidemiologist. When Welch was soliciting money from the Rockefeller Foundation to found the School of Hygiene and Public Health, it became apparent that a schism had arisen between public-health-oriented sanitarians, represented by Hermann Biggs and William Sedgwick, and academically oriented epidemiologists, individuals who did not yet exist except in the mind of Welch. That Frost kept one foot in the waters of public health while planting the other on the terrain of academia would do much to insure the future productive cooperation of the two related fields.

There was a long-standing linkage between the School of Hygiene and Public Health and the Rockefeller Foundation. Welch had secured the original funding and endowment for the school from the foundation. Indeed, he had offered to name the school for Rockefeller, an offer that was declined. Public health had been a major area of interest to the Rockefeller Foundation at its inception, and indeed, it has remained so to this day.

John D. Rockefeller was an extraordinary man.[48] A ruthless, aggressive, imaginative, and exceptionally successful businessman, he founded the Standard Oil Company and used it to monopolize the production and transport of petroleum products in North America and much of the world. His large holdings in the Standard Oil Company produced an income unparalleled in America. Rockefeller was also a religious man and one who devoted much of his time and energy to philanthropy, in part directed to his church, but mostly to education and science. In addition to Johns Hopkins University, Rockefeller or his foundation endowed Spellman College in Atlanta, the University of Chicago, the London School of Tropical Medicine and Hygiene, and the Rockefeller Institute for Medical Research, which later became Rockefeller University. Rockefeller's son, John D. Rockefeller Jr. devoted nearly full time simply to managing his father's philanthropic gifts.

As early as 1901, Rockefeller envisioned establishing a foundation for the purpose of distributing his benevolences. In 1909, he pledged 73,000 shares of Standard Oil stock, then worth about $50 million, for this purpose. In 1913, Rockefeller gave an additional $100 million, followed by a further $82.8 million six years later, when the foundation was chartered.[49] From its inception the Rockefeller Foundation made public health a focus of its activities. It took over the work of the Rockefeller Sanitary Commission, which had been founded in 1909 to combat hookworm infestations in the southern United States with a one million dollar gift from Rockefeller. Here were its roots in public health. It then established the Rockefeller International Health Commission (later renamed the International Division) to support public health efforts on a global scale.

From 1929 to 1932 Frost served a three-year term as a scientific director of the International Division of the Rockefeller Foundation. This was not a trivial appointment, for in this position he had a major impact on the expenditures of this large philanthropic organization. Frost's opinions were highly regarded, and he had a great influence on the International Division and its advisory board, which was chaired by Welch at that time. Decisions of this board sometimes were in conflict with the ideas of the foundation's director.[50]

Frost also worked with the Milbank Fund, first as a member of its advisory council in 1934, then as a member of its technical board in 1936. Frost's friend and colleague Edgar Sydenstricker had become the scientific director of the fund. Not surprisingly, Frost was a consultant to the New York State Health Department and to a number of other state and local health departments.

He received abundant recognition by his fellow scientists and sanitarians during his life. He was elected to the prestigious

Cosmos Club in Washington, D.C. Founded in 1878 by John Wesley Powell, the club became a meeting place for American intellectual leaders from many disciplines. During Frost's life, the club was sited in the Dolly Madison House on Lafayette Square. In 1938 the American Public Health Association awarded Frost the Sedgwick Memorial Medal, the association's highest honor and the most prestigious award in the field of public health. Frost was dying at the time, as his friends knew, and seemed unlikely to survive until the September meeting at which the medal was customarily presented. Therefore the medal was given to Frost in the hospital by his wife on April 11, 1938, a scant three weeks before his death. Posthumously, Frost was honored by many tributes and by the establishment of a named lectureship of the American Public Health Association and an endowed, named professorship at the University of Virginia Health Sciences Center.

10

Epidemiologist

Epidemiology at any given time is something
more than the total of its established facts.
— *Wade Hampton Frost*[1]

Wade Hampton Frost spent the last two decades of his life at
Johns Hopkins University in Baltimore. The first ten years of
his tenure there were largely devoted to launching the science
of epidemiology at Johns Hopkins and throughout the public
health and medical worlds of North America. He continued his
work on influenza and water pollution, an enduring interest of
his, and he remained a consultant to the United States Public
Health Service in the latter area even after he resigned his commission. Yet important, broader, and more fundamental ideas
were germinating in his fertile mind. During his second decade
in Baltimore, he made major contributions to his discipline.
They were not made in abstract or theoretical contexts. Rather,
they were anchored in investigations of major epidemic diseases. Fundamental and important papers came forth, often
coauthored with his students or junior faculty colleagues.
Some of the fundamental concepts and techniques he pioneered are known to the world principally through the works
of those to whom he taught them.

Ernest Stebbins, one of Frost's students in the early 1930s
and later dean of the Johns Hopkins School of Hygiene and
Public Health, reflected on Frost's interactions with his students
and junior colleagues vis-a-vis their research, interactions that
in the current world of science would almost certainly have
meant coauthorship of the resulting paper.

I'd have my tables and what I had drafted as a paper, and he would
go over it carefully, and he'd look for those jokers with you. Oh, he

devoted an awful lot of time to his students. . . . A number of papers that I wrote should have had his name on [them], because he did just as much as I did, but he wouldn't. . . . I would have been so proud to have his name on a paper with mine, but he said, "no, you did this research. I'm just reviewing it with you."[2]

Similarly, Miriam Brailey, who studied with Frost and then joined his faculty, acknowledged Frost in a footnote to a 1937 paper reporting her study of tuberculosis in children at the Harriet Lane Pediatric Tuberculosis Clinic, noting that he "directed the analysis of data from clinical records."[3] Surely, any professor who had contributed in such a manner would have been named as a coauthor on a publication today.

Frost resigned his Public Health Service commission in August 1929, ten years after joining the Johns Hopkins faculty on loan from the service. During that first decade he remained in charge of the Cincinnati field station, which had been reopened and reorganized late in 1919 after the conclusion of World War I. John K. Hoskins, a Public Health Service sanitary engineer, was appointed to be "in immediate charge." Frost traveled to Cincinnati as needed, and even after resigning his commission served as a consultant in stream pollution. In 1924 and 1926 he published detailed accounts of the status of water in the Ohio River and of the activities of the Public Health Service in studying water pollution.[4] Under his and Hoskins's leadership, the field station undertook frustrating and by-and-large unrewarding studies of the means by which stream water purified itself naturally. They hoped that comprehension of how flowing water cleansed itself would lead to better filtration techniques, but they were not able to unravel and understand nature's complex purification processes. Additionally, they surveyed sewage disposal and water purification plants along the Ohio River and its tributaries.

Frost's interests in water purity were not confined to the Ohio River and its tributaries. In 1925 Conrad Kinyoun, an Assistant Bacteriologist at the Hygienic Laboratory of the United States Public Health Service, published a study of oysters as possible vectors for typhoid fever.[5] Kinyoun purchased oysters from the

Chesapeake Bay that were being offered for sale to the public. He placed them in an aquarium jar with salt water, tested them for viability, and then added a culture of typhoid bacilli to the water in the aquarium jar. He then cultured the oysters over the next fifteen days, recovering typhoid organisms from them throughout that length of time. This result was not greeted cheerfully by Chesapeake Bay oystermen and vendors of oysters. The Surgeon General responded by appointing Frost to chair a committee to study the sanitary qualities of shell fish, focusing chiefly on oysters harvested in Chesapeake Bay, and also including the coastal waters of Rhode Island and Massachusetts. In this capacity Frost studied the problem in cooperation with representative of the Bureau of Chemistry, the Bureau of Fisheries, and the Oyster and Shellfish Association of America.

In 1925, 1926, and 1927, Frost represented the Public Health Service at conferences on water pollution and reported on findings of this committee.[6] The deliberations of the committee with its diverse representatives each with parochial interests were not always harmonious. At the 1928 conference Frost, unable to make a final report from the committee studying shell fish, noted that:

> There have been differences of opinion and prolonged debates between [committee] members as to what the bacteriological specifications [for safe human consumption] ought to be. . . . [However,] shellfish sold in the market [are], generally speaking, reasonably safe in so far as we can judge from present knowledge.[7]

There remained, for Frost, some unfinished reckonings of the 1918–1919 influenza epidemic, and he published two major reports dealing with this epidemic during his Johns Hopkins tenure. His first effort was devoted to looking at case incidence and case fatality rates.[8] As noted in chapter 7, Frost turned to household surveys conducted in selected communities, since accurate national data for this epidemic did not exist. In choosing this modality, he foreshadowed some of his later major studies of tuberculosis in which household surveys were used. The case rates documented in the chosen populations ranged from 150 to 535 per 1,000; that is, from 15 percent to more than 50 percent of all persons in those communities became ill with influenza during this great pandemic. It can be presumed that these high attack rates prevailed throughout North America and much of the world. While young children were most likely to become sick, deaths from influenza were most likely to occur in young adults and the elderly. This phenomenon, so well documented by Frost in this study, has been found to be present in subsequent major influenza epidemics.

Working as a consultant to his colleague and friend Edgar Sydenstricker and his associates (Sydenstricker was now in charge of the Office of Statistical Investigations of the Public Health Service in Washington) Frost helped to examine the mortality from influenza during the two-decade period spanning both sides of the great 1918–1919 epidemic.[9] The study was based on reported death data from fifty American cities, thirty-five of which provided the greatest detail in reported information. Monthly death rates were computed and rounded out to develop expected seasonal mortality curves. Excess deaths reported as due to pneumonia or influenza were then added to the curves to reveal the occurrence of epidemics of influenza at intervals of one to five years during the twenty-year study period. In general, excess death rates during these outbreaks peaked at about 200 per 100,000 and occurred in late winter—the first three months of the new year. When these figures were graphed, the 1918–1919 epidemic stood out in striking exception to all others. In October 1918, excess deaths reached nearly 4,800 per 100,000. In 1920, sixteen months after the peak of the major pandemic, excess mortality exceeded 1,200 per 100,000—a heartbreaking "after shock." Figure 10.1, reproduced from the published report, demonstrates with clarity the seasonal mortality peaks during years of influenza outbreaks. The technique of tracking influenza by noting excess pneumonia deaths in selected cities is still used, although it is now complemented by sentinel surveys based on viral cultures, which became possible in the second half of the twentieth century.

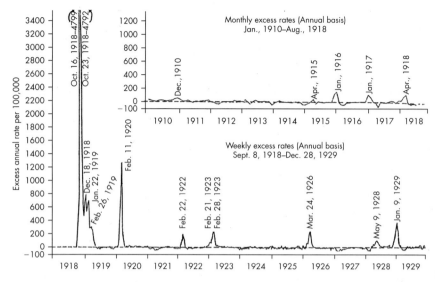

Figure 10.1. Excess influenza-pneumonia mortality in a group of 35 large cities in the United States, 1910–1929. Dates on graph are middle (Wednesday) of the peak weeks. (Prior to July 1, 1919, excess rates are deviations from the median rates 1910–1916; after that date they are deviations from the median rates 1921–1927.) Reproduced from Collins SD, Frost WH, Glover M, Sydenstricker E. Mortality from influenza and pneumonia in 50 large cities of the United States, 1910-1929. *Public Health Rep.* 1930;45:2277–329.

Frost's epidemiology curriculum at Johns Hopkins required a thesis of each student, and he needed to generate ideas for these projects. While some of these student efforts were limited in scope, important studies evolved from many of them. Given his background in influenza, it was natural for Frost to set his students working on acute respiratory infections. The first of these to come under his scrutiny was diphtheria. Diphtheria was a frightening disease that focused its ravages on children, in whom it was often fatal if not treated promptly with antiserum. Early in his public health career at the Hygienic Laboratory, Frost had studied the immunity conveyed by this serum. Many cases of diphtheria occurred in Baltimore each year, and one of Frost's first students, Reginald Atwater, was set to work studying the epidemiology of the disease as his thesis project. He was the first of four graduate students who devoted their theses to diphtheria under the tutelage of Frost. Additional studies of diphtheria were conducted under the leadership of James Doull. Others picked up the cudgel in later years.

In February 1928 Frost delivered two Cutter Lectures in Preventive Medicine at Harvard Medical School. For one of these he chose the topic, "Infection, Immunity and Disease in the Epidemiology of Diphtheria" (published later that year in the *Journal of Preventive Medicine*).[10] Frost reviewed the then current knowledge of the transmission of the toxin-producing bacterium that causes diphtheria and of host immunity to its toxin. This immune state could be recognized with a simple skin test developed earlier by Béla Schick in Vienna. Frost then noted that, "a negative Schick test, although it indicates immunity to the *disease,* does not imply immunity against *carrier-infection.*"[11] A carrier state exists for diphtheria, as it does for a number of infectious diseases. Frost recognized, perhaps for the first time, that this carrier state might confer immunity even in the absence of clinical disease. Thus, healthy individuals with negative Schick tests may reflect this immune carrier state. Moreover, Frost proposed, an apparent epidemic may be no more than a change in the ratio between persons carrying the bacillus asymptomatically and those who are ill. Frost reviewed data from Baltimore and elsewhere and concluded that this ratio varied geographically and could not be assumed to be an inherent property of the interactions between humans and this disease-causing bacillus. Perhaps, he hypothesized, populations with a large proportion of individuals immunized by frequent passage of bacteria among carriers were less often afflicted by outbreaks of diphtheria. More knowledge was needed, he concluded.

Schick had observed that children who had had tonsillectomies were more likely to manifest immunity to diphtheria toxin than those who had not had their tonsils removed when tested six weeks following the operation, presumably because the procedure stimulated the development of immunity. James Doull had confirmed this observation in Baltimore, although his data were less striking than Schick's. In 1931 Ralph Wheeler (one of Frost's graduate students), Doull, and Frost reported on the antidiphtheria toxin immunity of young adults who had or had not had tonsillectomy.[12] No differences were observed. Perhaps the immunity noted by Schick was not long lasting, they suggested.

In the mid 1930s Morton Levin, a student, took on a comparison of the status of diphtheria carrier states prevalent in Baltimore in 1921–1924 and 1933–1934 as the subject of his thesis. His studies led to a more complete report published in the American Journal of Hygiene in 1936.[13] Diphtheria had been declining in the United States since 1900, he noted, and the rate of decline greatly accelerated beginning in about 1927. With this decline, the case-fatality rate also declined. Only a few of the diphtheria bacilli one can culture from carriers are toxin producers. Frost, Levin, and their colleagues found that the toxin-producers fell from 2.44% in the winters of 1921–22 to 1.08% in the winter of 1934–36 (these numbers were lower than actual rates because of limitations in the bacteriologic techniques used). It appeared that the diphtheria bacilli in Baltimore had become less virulent. At the same time, the fraction of children whose Schick tests indicated immunity rose from 54.1% to 65.6%. Much of these changes the investigators attributed to the introduction of childhood vaccination against diphtheria, a practice that continues to the present—the D in DPT shots. Yet, as they analyzed their data and developed mathematical equations to refine this evaluation, the epidemiologists were forced to conclude that only part of the reduced morbidity and mortality was due to the introduction of vaccination. Either human resistance to diphtheria had increased or the virulence of the organism had decreased.

No one would dispute the notion that the common cold is the most frequent of all acute respiratory illnesses and that, while not a serious illness, it is a major health problem. In 1923, the Public Health Service began a longitudinal survey of the occurrence of colds as reported by a group of university students and faculty members and by medical officers of the armed forces and their families. Frost's friend Edgar Sydenstricker was the statistician working on this project. In collaboration

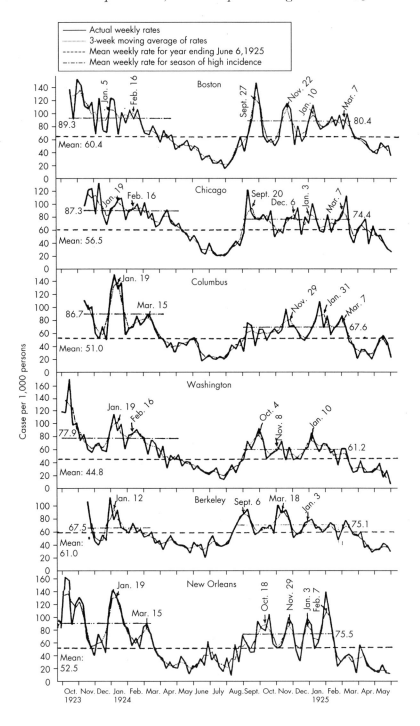

with Mary Gover, one of Sydenstricker's statisticians, Frost examined the occurrence of colds during several winter seasons.[14] Each peak of illness tended to last three to five weeks. As in figure 10.2, there was a surprising degree of synchrony between outbreaks within the winter season in various geographic locations. "It is truly remarkable," they wrote, "that . . . there should be such close correspondence between cities with respect to the time of occurrence of the epidemics."[15] They then noted that similar peaks of influenza occurred during highly prevalent years, although the influenza peaks tended to occur later in the winter season. This study was neither the first nor would it be the last longitudinal observation study of a defined population group. However, it set a high standard for work of this type.

Unable to explain the peaks of common colds, Frost remained intrigued, and he assigned the problem to one of his graduate students, Vivian Van Valkenburgh, who joined the Department of Epidemiology faculty after receiving his degree in 1929 and continued to work on common colds during the ensuing half-dozen years. Van Valkenburgh set about following 562 members of 114 Baltimore families from November 1928 to November 1930. The attack rate during the first twelve months was 318 colds per 100 persons observed (an average of 3.18 colds in each person); for the second year it was 307 colds per 100 persons observed.[16] That these rates were essentially the same was remarkable, for a major influenza outbreak occurred during the first year whereas influenza was nearly absent from Baltimore during the second year. The two respiratory infections were totally independent of one another.

Figure 10.2. Case incidence (weekly rates) of all respiratory affections, exclusive of hay fever, among college student groups reporting semimonthly to the United States Public Health Service, October 1923, to May 1935, in six cities. Reproduced from Frost WH, Gover M. The incidence and time distribution of common colds in several groups kept under continuous observation. *Public Health Rep.* 1932; 47:1815–41.

A closer look was clearly needed and it was soon forthcoming.[17] The findings from the 114 families and a subgroup of 88 for which the data were more complete were reviewed and analyzed. It was then possible to distinguish influenza from common colds in these families and show that each presented its separate and distinct epidemiologic pattern of occurrence during the winter season. On the basis of these epidemiological studies and without culture techniques, which were not known at the time, Frost concluded that separate epidemic waves of the common cold are caused by different viruses; that is, that there is not a single cold virus but many.

An interesting coda to Frost's interest in the common cold was played at the University of Virginia, Frost's alma mater. When that institution created an endowed Wade Hampton Frost Professorship of Medicine, it chose Jack M. Gwaltney Jr. for the position. Gwaltney, who had been trained in both epidemiology and virology, had an international reputation as the leading expert on the common cold and the transmission of viruses causing it. The University of Virginia studies conducted by Gwaltney and his colleagues, done when viral isolation methods had become available, confirmed Frost's hypothesis that the different peaks of illness were due to different families of cold viruses.

These studies of diphtheria and the common cold were more than simply refinements of prior observations of a well-known diseases. They added a great deal of knowledge about the natural history of the carrier state of diphtheria and the seasonal occurrence of colds. However, there is a more transcendent value to this body of work. What Frost and his colleagues did in these studies was to use the quantitative tools of epidemiology—this new science that they were inventing—to add to our understanding of certain infectious diseases. True, so did the pioneering work of Budd on typhoid, Snow on cholera, and Panum on measles. So also did Frost's investigations of polio. But beginning with Frost's studies of influenza, and continuing with his and his coworkers' investigations of diphtheria and common colds, quantification and mathematical analyses were introduced that had been lacking from all of the earlier work. Epidemiologists of today measure the effects they study; Frost taught them how to do so.

During these years at Johns Hopkins, Frost's reputation grew. He was repeatedly sought as a speaker or contributor to compendia, and he used many of these opportunities to discuss his views of the nature of epidemiology, the role of epidemiologists, and the contributions his science could make to the health of the public. He repeatedly called for scientific rigor among his academic peers, public health colleagues, and fellow epidemiologists.

Addressing the American Public Health Association in 1924, Frost considered the differences in the demands the public made for accounting of its money and the demands science placed upon the public health officer. For example, he noted that the public might be well pleased when a new water purification system was followed by a decrease in the occurrence of typhoid fever. However, Frost noted, a scientific public health officer must use statistical analysis to demonstrate that the observed decline in disease was significant. But that would not be sufficient to demonstrate causality. The next step in reasoning should be to consider whether similar measures have had similar results in other water purification instances. Finally, the rigorous public health officer must marshal all of the known facts of the epidemiology of typhoid fever and be certain that the outcome is consistent with these known facts. What Frost was doing in expounding the merits of this analysis was enjoining his listeners to be sure that no other factor of the type he liked to call a "joker," a "confounding variable" in the parlance of modern savants of epidemiology, was involved in the outcome. He then noted that periodic medical inspection of school children had been widely adopted in American cities. However, he commented, "I am not aware that anyone has even attempted as yet to demonstrate the ultimate effect of this work."[18]

In 1936, once again addressing the American Public Health Association, Frost considered the major functions of the society, noting that there were two.[19] The first of these was to provide members with the opportunity to exchange information with

their colleagues through meetings and the publication of a journal. Frost considered that function well served and without difficulties. The second activity of the society was to develop
standards and uniform procedures and express them as authoritative opinions, an activity being carried out by committees of
the society. Frost felt there was reason for concern in this area,
however—"a real and constant danger that [these] authoritative
pronouncements [might not be] based on adequate evidence."
Here we see Frost functioning as a senior statesman in the society and in the field of public health, cautioning those who would
neglect the need for scientific rigor in the name of expediency.

The following year Frost, in the role of "elder statesman,"
again spoke out at the meeting of the American Public Health
Association.[20] Speaking on epidemiology in a session devoted
to the topic, "What Every Health Officer Should Know," he
noted that "the most important preparation in epidemiology is
not any particular amount and kind of knowledge but the
desire, the determination and ability to add to it." He challenged health officers to learn of the origins of specific preventive measures and to know upon what evidence their presumed
efficacy was based. He urged them to read the works of "the
old masters of epidemiology:"

> It seems to me especially instructive to read the best of the public
> health literature of the latter part of the 19th century. The events and
> the thoughts are not too remote from our own and there has been
> sufficient time to uncover a good many of the errors and to confirm
> the conclusions which were correct.
>
> Such reading should serve the double purpose of cultivating dis-
> criminating judgement of scientific evidence and reasoning and of
> revealing to the health officer of today the opportunities which lie
> before him for useful investigations which he himself may undertake
> to carry through, opportunities which perhaps he has failed to
> perceive because they are so commonplace. For it is surprising how
> much of basic evidence in epidemiology has been derived from well
> ordered, simple observation in the small field encompassed by a local
> health officer or a country practitioner.[21]

At the same association meeting, the last he attended, Frost
spoke of the importance of classifying cases of the same disease

occurring within the same family as primary or secondary cases.[22] Once again, he revealed his respect for early work in the field, and he cited Charles V. Chapin, Superintendent of Health for Providence, Rhode Island, from 1884 to 1905, as the originator of the concept. In fact, however, Peter Ludwig Panum had clearly understood this concept when he investigated epidemic measles on the Faroe Islands in 1846.[23] Frost knew Panum's work, for he had commissioned its translation into English and had used it in his teaching, but he appears to have overlooked it in his 1937 address. If data are carefully recorded, making the distinction between primary and secondary cases, Frost noted, would allow the calculation of a secondary attack rate, which he defined as

> the risk of attack borne by others in the same household within specified periods of time, and how does this risk vary with the character and management of the original case and with the sex, age, past history, and various other circumstances of those exposed.[24]

Frost couched his mathematically and epidemiologically-oriented concepts in practical terms that surely had meaning for every district health officer in his audience.

Despite his enormous interest in the techniques of epidemiology as a scientific discipline as reflected in his teaching, Frost wrote only a single textbook chapter. In 1928 he contributed a chapter to a multiauthored text edited by Haven Emerson at Columbia University.[25] Emerson had been New York City's health commissioner in 1916 when Frost had investigated polio in that city. Frost devoted the first fourth of his chapter to reviewing the history of his discipline. He then turned his attention to the general characteristics of epidemics of infectious diseases, and concluded:

> There appear to be two general laws of epidemics; first, that infection tends to increase progressively, due to multiplication of foci; and second, that it is progressively checked by the resultant decrease in susceptibles, due to specific immunizations and deaths in the host population.[26]

As noted in the chapter 9, Frost was thinking at this time about a mathematical expression of the epidemic curve. Very likely this line of thought had been stimulated by his interactions and joint teaching with Lowell Reed, and the ultimate expression of this reasoning was a product of the two men. Merrell states that Frost "laid the theoretical ground work" and that Reed "refined the statistical aspects."[27] Frost's text chapter quoted from above is the only publication, during his lifetime, of this major contribution to the fundamental underpinnings of epidemiology. As noted previously, he did draft a manuscript that was edited and published nearly four decades after his death.[28]

The final fourth of Frost's text chapter is devoted to the epidemiology of specific diseases. As he did so often in his teaching, he drew his examples from classic historical studies, using John Snow's investigations of cholera to illustrate his points.

Frost's greatest contributions both to the understanding of a specific disease and to the field of epidemiology came from his studies of tuberculosis. That he waited until his second decade at Johns Hopkins to undertake these studies is remarkable. Not only had the importance of this affliction been made real to him by his own bout with the Captain of Death, but others in his family had also died or suffered from tuberculosis. Additionally, tuberculosis was a major health problem of the United States and Baltimore. In 1920, tuberculosis ranked third among causes of deaths registered in the United States, trailing only "other diseases" and heart disease. In 1930 tuberculosis ranked number six in the deadly roster, following heart disease, cancer, nephritis, pneumonia, and violent and accidental deaths.[29] Specific tuberculosis mortality data for geographic regions of special interest to Frost are given in table 10.1. (For comparison, it may be of interest that in the year 2000 there were only 751 deaths due to tuberculosis in the United States.[30]) Surely, many of Frost's students would have to deal with the white plague as they took up public health posts.

What deterred Frost from studying tuberculosis? One must realize that collecting data for a chronic infectious disease, for an epidemic with a periodic cycle perhaps measured in

Table 10.1
Tuberculosis mortality statistics for 1920 and 1930 for the United States, Baltimore, Maryland, and Tennessee given as number of deaths from all forms of tuberculosis in the registration area. Data for this table are taken from the annual mortality statistics reports of the United States Department of Commerce, Bureau of the Census.

	1920	1930
United States*	99,916	84,741
Baltimore	1,105	975
Maryland	2,139	1,721
Tennessee	3,860	3,132

*The national registration area in 1920 included 34 states, the District of Columbia, and sixteen cities in nonregistration area states, and comprised an estimated 90 percent of the population. In 1930 it included all states except Texas, the District of Columbia, two territories, and eight cities in Texas and comprised 96.2 percent of the population.

centuries rather than years, is a daunting task. For tuberculosis the problem is further compounded by the fact that only about 5 percent of those infected with the tubercle bacillus become ill with recognizable disease. Thus, whatever interest in tuberculosis Frost might have had, it was much easier to study acute infections, and acute infections made much better topics for study by his students.

In the end, however, it was his students who led Frost into the fertile field of the study of tuberculosis. Many of them had been health officers in their communities before coming to Johns Hopkins to undertake a degree program there. Others planned careers as health officers. As noted, tuberculosis was a major public health problem in the United States at that time, and it ranked high on the problem list of every local health department. No fewer than fourteen student theses written with Frost's guidance were devoted to tuberculosis (see table 9.2). Some of Frost's students were destined to achieve distinction in the nation's public health campaign against the dread disease.

The pediatric unit of Johns Hopkins Hospital had been named for Harriet Lane, its benefactor. Edwards Park, the chief of this pediatric service and a professor of pediatrics, had an interest in tuberculosis in children. In 1928 he organized the Harriet

Lane Tuberculosis Clinic. Miriam Brailey, a 1930 graduate of the Johns Hopkins Medical School, entered the School of Hygiene and Public Health following her graduation from the medical school and earned her graduate degree in 1931. Her thesis was based on a review of patient records from the Harriet Lane Tuberculosis Clinic. She then joined the school's epidemiology department as its first woman faculty member, continuing to conduct her studies and treat children with tuberculosis at the Harriet Lane Clinic. From 1932 to 1941, Brailey served as the director of that clinic, and in 1941, she became the director of the Bureau of Tuberculosis of the Baltimore City Health Department. It was Brailey who conducted the long-term research at the Harriet Lane Clinic, and it was she who shepherded Hopkins' students through its examining rooms and file cabinets.[31] But Frost was never far removed from the work by Brailey and her students work at the clinic.

The Harriet Lane Clinic provided a remarkable laboratory for the study of childhood tuberculosis. Children less than two years old who were either known to be infected with tubercle bacilli because of a positive tuberculin skin test or who were at great risk because they lived in a home with an infectious patient were admitted to the clinic and followed carefully. Brailey and her students, with statistical help from Frost, were able to demonstrate that mortality in this group was very high—thirty-nine deaths from tuberculosis among 223 children in the first eight years—especially in the first year of life and that among African American infants it was triple that of the Caucasian children.[32] Demonstrating these findings was not as simple as it would seem, however. In Brailey's mind it was apparent that the death rate for the *first* year could be expressed as a simple percentage. For subsequent years, however, the number of individuals under observation would not be the same and could be expected to diminish as time went on.[33] For analyses in this circumstance it was necessary to use life table methods, and Frost and Lowell Reed, who together had devised major improvements in this statistical approach, provided the expertise that Brailey needed. Indeed, it is likely that Frost actually performed the statistical manipulations. If not, he certainly must have intimately supervised Brailey as she undertook the use of the newly devised methods.

A major location—an epidemiological laboratory, in fact—in which Frost and his students undertook to study tuberculosis was developed in Baltimore's Eastern Health District, which Frost had been instrumental in bringing into Johns Hopkins' public health fold. In 1933, 1936, and again in 1937 health department nurses and Johns Hopkins students conducted detailed health censuses of the fifteen thousand families living in the district by door-to-door canvassing. Building upon this base, a series of Frost's graduate students did their thesis work in the Eastern Health District. The first of these students was James Perkins, who earned his degree in 1933 and went on to a distinguished career as the leader of the National Tuberculosis Association, the first American voluntary health agency. Others included Charles Eller (1934), Alexander Gilliam (1934), Floyd M. Feldman (1935), Robert Dyar (1938), Carl Barkhaus (1938), and John Phair (1938).

It has always been true that students lead their teachers to new challenges, often to life-changing epiphanies. Yet the questioning student cannot do this alone; the teacher must have both a prepared and a receptive mind. So it was that Eugene Lindsay Bishop led his teacher, Wade Hampton Frost, to the arena of the latter's most important work. Bishop was born in Nashville, Tennessee, in 1886. He attended Vanderbilt University, where he earned his M.D. degree in 1914. In 1918 he went to work for the State Board of Health of Tennessee as the director of its rural sanitation programs. Seeking greater knowledge of his chosen field, he entered the Johns Hopkins School of Hygiene and Public Health in 1922 and received the school's Certificate in Public Health in 1923 (equivalent of the modern Master of Public Health degree). There, he found in Frost an inspiring teacher. Bishop returned to Tennessee following completion of his Johns Hopkins studies and was made Assistant Commissioner of Public Health (and also joined the faculty of Vanderbilt University in the department of public health). The following year he became the state's public health commissioner, serving in this post until 1935.

Tuberculosis was a major public health problem in Tennessee at that time. Although mortality rates were declining, the Tennessee tuberculosis death rate in relation to population size was consistently double that of the United States as a whole (numbers of tuberculosis deaths in Tennessee for 1920 and 1930 are given in table 10.1). Thus, Bishop felt that this disease needed his attention. With a grant from the Rosenwald Fund, Bishop established a study based on tuberculosis data available in Trenton, the county seat of Gibson County located in western Tennessee about eighty-five miles northeast of Memphis. The study began in 1930, and within a short time Bishop realized that the problem was more complex than he had envisioned. He turned to his teacher, Frost, for help and met with him on July 10, 1930. Frost reviewed Bishop's data with his characteristic thoroughness and then gave the younger man his advice: "The basic material for the study should be an unselected series of cases of tuberculosis." Frost then outlined in detail the extensive clinical and social histories that should be recorded for each tuberculosis case and for each household contact. And, he noted, it would be desirable to include a group of control households.[34]

Bishop was eager to take his mentor's advice. Much later he would write to Susan Frost, his professor's widow:

> Dr. Frost was more to me than a teacher—even more than a friend— for he represented an ideal which has inspired me in all the years since I had my graduate work under his guidance. No man whom I have ever known possesses in the same degree his qualities of intellect, nor his high personal attributes.[35]

Bishop and Frost concluded that it would be best to initiate a second study with a very different design, a design that certainly came from Frost's mind. Frost envisioned following a group of families over a period of time, much as he and his colleagues had been doing in their studies of acute respiratory illnesses in Baltimore. A study of this type could reveal the risk of tuberculous infection to persons in household contact with infectious cases. However, studying families for the occurrence of tuberculosis would be much more difficult than studying acute respiratory infections, for, in Frost's words, "the disease is of slow evolution, and we cannot assume that the risk with which we are concerned is concentrated within the year or even the decade following the establishment of the known exposure."[36] Studies would have to be long term. Bishop was excited by Frost's proposals, and aided by Frost he obtained funds to support the project from the International Division of the Rockefeller Foundation, of which Frost was then one of the scientific directors. Bishop and Frost selected Kingsport, Sullivan County, in Eastern Tennessee for the project. Because tuberculosis rates were higher in African Americans than Caucasians, they decided to carry out the study in African American families, all of which residing within the county were asked to participate. One hundred and thirty-two families joined the study; only three declined.

With respect to knowledge of tuberculosis, the major finding of the Kingsport study provided the first quantitative measurement of the risk of tuberculosis in family contact with diseased persons. When the risks were calculated using life table methods, the risk of tuberculosis expressed as an attack rate was 1.3% for those from tuberculous households as compared with 0.7% for those with no known family contact. The respective risks of death from tuberculosis were 0.5% and 0.2%. Living in a house with someone who had tuberculosis doubled one's risk of developing and of dying from the disease.[37]

Within a year of initiating the Kingsport study, Bishop and Frost had raised their sights and were planning a much more ambitious investigation of the natural history of tuberculosis. With continuing support from the Rockefeller Foundation, they decided to take on a household study of all of the cases of the disease occurring in Williamson County, Tennessee. Williamson County was a rural, largely agricultural county located south of Nashville. Its population was approximately twenty-five thousand. The study would not be a trivial one. In fact, during the twenty-four years of the study, 828 households were investigated, and more than thirty-two thousand person-years of observations were recorded.[38]

Existing epidemiological techniques were not adequate for the challenges these Tennessee studies posed. In refining existing methods and developing novel ones, Frost made some of his most important contributions to his discipline and laid the ground work for some of his later major contributions. There were three important methodological advances that came out of the Tennessee tuberculosis studies: (1) the concept of the index case, (2) modifications and applications of the life-table method, especially with respect to estimating secondary attack rates, and (3) the use of age cohorts in longitudinal studies.

With the discovery of a person ill with tuberculosis, health care workers entered the household and interviewed all of its members. Often times it was found that there had been an earlier individual in the home who, in fact, represented the beginning of a chain of infection. Yet there was one of Frost's "jokers" hidden in investigation of mortality rates of the contacts of this earliest source case, for the person who had actually first presented to the health department had defined himself or herself as not having died—at least not yet—as a result of the contact. To deal with this and related phenomena, Frost enunciated the concept of the "index case," a terminology now familiar to all who work in public health but entirely new at the time. The index case was the person who first came to attention, not necessarily the first person in the household to have tuberculosis.[39] Unbiased mortality risks could be calculated in the contacts of the index case. The use of the index case has become so fundamental to all epidemiological investigations, whether for research protocols or for disease control programs, that it is hard to believe it was not understood prior to Frost's elaboration of it in the Tennessee studies. Yet that was the case.

In any study conducted over time, some study subjects drop out for a variety of reasons. Perhaps they move away, perhaps they decline further interviews, perhaps they die of the disease being studied or of another cause. In short-term studies these drop-outs may not have an important impact on the results, but in a long-term study nothing can be made of the observations unless the drop-outs are dealt with. Over many years, initially in Europe including some studies of tuberculosis in British sanatoria, later in North America, statisticians had developed a technique known as the "life table" method in which the year-to-year risk is calculated with readjustment of the population size each year. In the end, person-years are used as denominators. Frost developed a straightforward tabular method for making these calculations in relation to age and demonstrated that the risk of mortality varied greatly with the age of the patient. In fact, in Kingsport the risk of dying from all causes for a child in family contact with tuberculosis during the first year of life was 5.19%; the same risk at age four to five was only 1.02%, and for an individual between forty and forty-nine years old it was 0.13%. These rates were substantially lower than those reported for African Americans in the rest of the state, possibly reflecting the relative affluence of this particular population. However, Frost noted, there might have been a substantial under-reporting of African American deaths in other Tennessee communities not under study.[40] Moreover, as noted below, one of Frost's "jokers" was at play here, for survival of the index case to the time of reporting was inherent in the Kingsport study data but not in the state statistics.

Prior to these Tennessee studies, a number of epidemiologists had looked at their findings by age cohorts and made cross-sectional comparisons of events occurring at different ages in this manner. In Frost's words, "these studies . . . must be carried out in *longitudinal section* rather than in *cross section*."[41] Reflecting on this work in 2002, George Comstock, Professor Emeritus of Epidemiology at Johns Hopkins, considered it to be the first use of age cohorts for longitudinal epidemiological studies.[42] Frost would make further refinements of this approach, and it would later serve as the basis for some of his most unique and original work.

The methodological advances made by Frost in the Tennessee studies of tuberculosis have been elegantly reviewed by Comstock. With respect to life-table analyses, they were first applied to the study of tuberculosis by Lawrason Brown, the eminent phthisiologist and disciple of Edward Livingston Trudeau at Saranac Lake in 1904. This method was largely forgotten by students of tuberculosis epidemiology thereafter. Frost rediscovered it and applied it to the Kingsport data. In Comstock's words,

> To avoid the long period of observation needed to study the future experience of a currently identified cohort, Frost hit upon the non-concurrent prospective or historical cohort approach. In essence, this involved interviewing a family informant and recording 3 sets of data: the date of establishment of each household, a list of all persons currently in each household and pertinent study information, and a list of former members of each household with pertinent study information. After reconstructing the cohort backward in time, Frost wisely decided to check its mortality experience by a person-years analysis, comparing age-specific mortality rates with those of the black population of Tennessee. His study cohort was found to have unexpectedly low death rates in the age group 20–49 years. Frost eventually found that the "joker" . . . was the fact that there had to be a living informant to provide information about a household, where as this was not true for the general population. . . . Although Frost [gave] credit to [others], his slightly different presentation of data and his failure to recognize that his joker was analogous to those of the earlier studies . . . make one wonder if Frost did not develop the person-time method independently and only later realize that their life table methods . . . were essentially the same as his.[43]

Not only does Comstock credit Frost with putting life-table methods on the tuberculosis epidemiology map, but he also points out that the Kingsport study was Frost's first use of longitudinal studies of age cohorts, thus laying the intellectual basis for some of his later major contributions.

The third of the Tennessee tuberculosis studies was conducted in Williamson County south of Nashville. Here Bishop, the former student, and Frost, the professor, planned a study based on reported cases with the objectives of elucidating the concurrent, antecedent, and subsequent manifestations of tuberculous infection and disease as determined by tuberculin skin testing, clinical histories and examinations, and radiographic examinations of all household members. These objectives immediately defined a project of large scope, especially when one realizes that the study was continued without interruption for twenty-four years. Nor were significant changes made in the program of work during those years, for Frost and Bishop had planned well, and Frost kept up his contact with the Williamson County investigators, traveling there at least semiannually. That Frost was, in fact, the major architect of this investigation was made clear in the final summary monograph published in 1963.[44]

The results of the study were published in nineteen scientific papers and two books as well as the summary monograph cited above. Sadly, Frost did not live to see most of them. Among the most important findings were data on the length of time between infection and the onset of disease. Prior thought in the scientific phthisiology community was that disease followed infection within the first few years or not at all. That this was incorrect was clearly demonstrated in this longitudinal study of more than two decades duration. Moreover, the interval between infection and onset of disease was strongly influenced by the age at which infection occurred.[45] Infants and young adults tended to develop disease rather promptly; school-aged children tended to control their infection until the post puberty years of adolescence and young adulthood. This observation is well illustrated in figure 10.3.

Age was not the only factor influencing the development of tuberculosis. Genes played a role as well. Attack rates in young Caucasian adults with a blood relationship to the index case were twice the rates when there was no blood relationship to the index case (results were limited to this ethnic and age group because only in this group were the numbers sufficient to allow analysis).[46] Race played some role, but not a major one. African Americans were found to have similar risks of infection and disease from their household contacts with the germ, but the extent of pulmonary disease they developed was frequently greater than that seen in Caucasians.[47] These concepts were not new, but the Tennessee study put them on firm, statistically valid ground.

One of the great conceptual tenets of the medical community interested in tuberculosis was crumbling at the time of the Williamson County study, and the Tennessee investigators contributed to its demise. Since the early work of Clemens

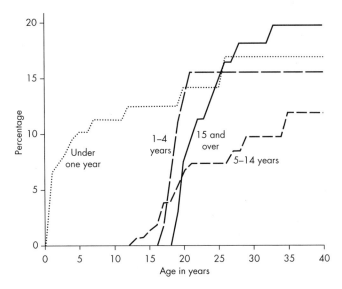

Figure 10.3. Cumulative probability per 100 of developing tuberculosis, by age, for children of index cases with sputum positive for acid-fast bacilli [tubercle bacilli—TMD], according to age at first exposure, Williamson County Tuberculosis Study. Figure from Zeidberg LD, Dillon A, Gass RS. Risk of developing tuberculosis among children of tuberculous parents. *Am Rev Tuberc.* 1954; 70:1008–19. Reproduced with permission.

von Pirquet, a positive tuberculin test was taken to indicate tuberculous infection with great sensitivity and specificity. However, it was becoming apparent that many individuals with apparent tuberculosis revealed by chest roentgenograms had negative tuberculin skin tests. From many studies, including the Williamson County study, it became evident that these tuberculin-negative, radiograph-positive persons actually had histoplasmosis, a usually benign pulmonary infection caused by a soil fungus widely prevalent in the central United States.[48]

The Williamson County study was the most ambitious of the three investigations initiated by Bishop in Tennessee with Frost's guidance and counsel. The Gibson County and Kingsport studies were more modest. The follow-up interval in Kingsport was a manageable 7.5 years, while the Williamson County study lasted nearly a quarter of a century. As it continued, the contributions of the Vanderbilt University faculty increased, without diminishing the antecedent influence of Frost and others at Johns Hopkins. In the monograph giving the final summary report of the project, twenty-seven investigators and consultants were acknowledged; seven of them were faculty colleagues or had been students of Frost at Johns Hopkins.

The Tennessee tuberculosis studies made important contributions to epidemiological methodology. They also contributed to our knowledge of the natural history of tuberculosis, then and now a disease of great importance throughout the inhabited world. They upset prior theories that had grown out of experience with patients in tuberculosis sanatoria, an experience biased by the advanced nature of the disease in most sanatorium patients. Furthermore, the Tennessee studies had a major impact on Frost's thinking about tuberculosis. He understood, perhaps more clearly than any other person of the era, that the natural history of tuberculosis and the epidemiology of the disease were inseparably intertwined. In an address delivered in 1935 at a symposium during the Thirty-First Annual Meeting of the National Tuberculosis Association in Saranac Lake, New York, Frost commented that it is unreasonable to hope that transmission of the disease from person to person could be completely prevented by public health measures. Yet, he noted, tuberculosis mortality had been declining in the United States for at least fifty years. All that was necessary, he posited, was that transmission be reduced and kept below the level at which a given number of infectious individuals transmit their disease to a sufficient number of susceptible persons to carry on the succession. That is, Frost argued, in order to survive, the tubercle bacillus requires a surplus of chances to establish new infections in susceptible persons.[49] With an aggressive public health program, tuberculosis might be eradicated in North America, Frost suggested, but he cautioned against raising public hopes unless the requisite control measures were firmly in place. The importance of Frost's comments at this time lies not in his call for a strong tuberculosis control program but in the fact that he clearly recognized that the tuberculosis epidemic was on the wane, irrespective of human intervention. Two years later after once again expressing caution that it was necessary to maintain an effective program of tuberculosis control, he opined "that under present conditions . . . the tubercle bacillus is losing ground, and . . . the eventual eradication of tuberculosis requires only that the present balance against it be maintained."[50]

Frost's greatest contribution to an understanding of the natural history of tuberculosis was made during the last few years of his life. Working with data from Massachusetts provided to him by Edgar Sydenstricker, Frost began to look at tuberculosis mortality by age cohort. He wished

> to call attention to the apparent change in age selection which has taken place gradually during the last 30 to 60 years, and to note that when looked at from a different point of view this change in age selection is found to be more apparent than real.[51]

Tuberculosis was known to be a disease of young adults. That fact was well established by centuries of experience and was clearly demonstrated in the Tennessee tuberculosis studies. However, as decades had rolled past during the late nineteenth and early twentieth centuries, tuberculosis in the United States looked more and more like a disease of the elderly. The Massachusetts data clearly showed this change. What Frost realized was that some of the individuals of a given cohort, say that cohort born in the 1880s, escaped from the young adult mortality that hit the cohort at the turn of the century when its members were in their twenties. Those escapees lived on, but broke down with active tuberculosis later in life. Looking at the cohort born in the 1910s, Frost noted that its members also had their peak mortality as young adults in the 1930s. However, rapidly declining tuberculosis infection incidences in the United States meant that the young adult peak of tuberculosis incidence for this later cohort, although clearly a peak, was lower than the incidence of disease in the earlier cohort, now in its fifth decade of life and past its early adult peak. This cohort's disease, now more frequent than the disease of younger persons, was a legacy of its past infections. The sum of these various age cohorts produced a trend in which the young adult peak was steadily diminishing and in which late life disease peaks were steadily increasing. This concept is illustrated in figure 10.4, taken from Frost's paper. In Frost's words in a 1935 letter to Sydenstricker:

> Viewed in this light the relatively high mortality rates now exhibited in the higher age groups [should] be interpreted as the residuum of the much higher rates which the now aged cohorts have experienced in earlier life.[52]

Frost worked on his concepts for several years, beginning in the early 1930s. He first presented his observations to the Southern Branch of the American Public Health Association in 1936. He became ill the following year and died before submitting this paper for publication. He left a final draft, however, and his Johns Hopkins colleagues submitted it to the

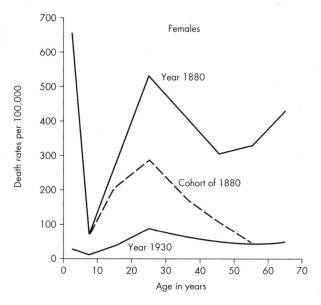

Figure 10.4. Massachusetts death rates for women from tuberculosis—all forms—by age, in the years 1880 and 1930 and for the cohort of 1880. Frost's dotted line for the 1880 cohort makes it clear that disease in this cohort was largely responsible for the late life peak observed in the year 1930. Figure from Frost WH. The age selection of mortality from tuberculosis in successive decades. *Am J Hyg.* 1939; 30:91–96. Reproduced with permission.

American Journal of Hygiene where it was published in 1939. It was immediately recognized as a seminal piece of work, probably, in the view of George Comstock, because of "Frost's ability to express his reasoned conclusions in readily understood language."[53]

In his paper Frost cited the work of Kristian Andvord, a Norwegian epidemiologist who had reviewed mortality in European countries.[54] Published in Norwegian in 1930 and shortly thereafter in German, Andvord's analysis reached much the same conclusion that Frost's did. One then must ask how original Frost's work was and whether he did more than copy the methods of Andvord. In fact, it is quite apparent that Frost's ideas germinated well before he knew of Andvord's work. Frost's papers archived at Johns Hopkins University include tables and graphs of tuberculosis mortality data for 1901, 1910, and 1911 for various North American cities.[55] Unfortunately, these documents are not dated. The Kingsport data are tabulated in this way as well, and, as noted, Frost had emphasized the need for longitudinal surveillance of age cohorts to his colleagues in Tennessee in memoranda in 1930 and 1931. In 1932 he discussed the use of cohorts with James Perkins, one of his students at the time.[56] Also, in the Johns Hopkins archives are tabulations of data from the Russian steppes taken from a paper by Elie Metchnikoff and others published in 1911;[57] Frost organized these data by age cohorts. Finally, it should be noted that in the 1935 letter to his friend and colleague, Edgar Sydenstricker, asking him to review an early draft of his manuscript, he made no mention of Andvord's work.[58] In fact, in this letter, he noted, *"For some years* [emphasis added] I have thought of the high mortality in later life as being related to *escape* from excessive mortality in earlier adult life."[59] George Comstock, the modern dean of tuberculosis epidemiologists and a student of Frost's life and work, believes that Frost was thinking about the form of analysis that led to his pioneering paper for several years and that he became aware of Andvord's work only after he had prepared a late draft of his paper.[60]

How then does Frost's analysis compare with that of Andvord? They both had the same general idea, but Frost's exposition is clearer and states its conclusions in a more straightforward fashion. His graphic representations are more readily understood than Andvord's. Without diminishing the importance of the early Norwegian work, it was Frost's paper that had the major impact upon our modern understanding of the epidemiology of the waning phase of the great tuberculosis epidemic of North America and Europe.

Progressing from relatively straightforward studies of acute infectious diseases to the exceedingly complex investigation of chronic infectious ailments, Frost's two decades of epidemiological studies at Johns Hopkins were marked by a series of major contributions both to the understanding of the nature of major infectious diseases and to the methods needed to acquire that understanding. Few others—perhaps no others – have contributed so much in this field. Moreover, Frost accomplished much of this by empowering his students, and his legacy continued long after a premature death withdrew this remarkable man from the lists.

11

Sunset and Evening Star

> There are things above all that all men most
> admire in others and most want for themselves,
> courage to fight to the last ditch against all odds,
> and courage to die bravely if the fight is lost.
> —*Wade Hampton Frost*[1]

As winter crept into Baltimore in late 1937, it became apparent that Wade Hampton Frost was not well. He was troubled with abdominal pain, and he had difficulty swallowing. He was losing weight. In January 1938 he cancelled a planned visit to his daughter in Boston because of chest pain. Soon it became evident that he had cancer of his esophagus. Even today that cancer is one that is hard to eradicate, and for Frost there was not much hope. Ironically, it was epidemiological methodology, much of it pioneered by Frost, that would later establish the link between this form of cancer and cigarettes, to which Frost was addicted.

As the illness progressed, Frost spent increasing lengths of time in the hospital. Several poignant letters written by Frost to his wife from his hospital bed survive, but are not dated. One appears to have been written at a time when a biopsy or other tests had been performed and he was awaiting the results from Louis Hamman, a leading Johns Hopkins clinician who was apparently one of Frost's attending physicians. Its accepting, almost fatalistic tone is similarly present in the other surviving letters; it is revealing of Frost's mental state as his illness progressed.

Thursday a.m.

Dearest—

There isn't any news, of course, and if there were, Dr. Baker would have phoned you, as I presume he has done in any case.

Yesterday was pretty well taken up with examinations of one kind and another, including several X-ray[s], and a visit to Dr. Crowe—all rather pestiferous but not painful. Though I still have my bellyache at times, I've been fairly comfortable here, and certainly have not lacked the most considerate attention from everybody . . . .

I presume Dr. Hamman will come in today or tomorrow and that then or soon thereafter he'll be ready to write my prescription[. F]or the present it is just day to day.

I wrote you a scrawl last night which Miss Collins (the head nurse) said she would give to you instead of mailing it, as she expected you this p.m. It seems silly for me not to see you if you come.

Best love,

Jack[2]

Wade Hampton Frost died on May 1, 1938, a scant two months after his fifty-eighth birthday. His passing was marked by many obituaries and tributes. John Owens, editor-in-chief of the *Baltimore Sun* and a close friend of Frost, wrote, in part:

One of the fine and rare spirits passed from this earth on Sunday morning. . . . To his work his associates will give tribute in due course. But . . . those who knew him well . . . will think: Wherever he stood, there knighthood remained in flower.

He had a deep wisdom for the affairs of life, and he had a subtle and penetrating wit. He had an austere sense of duty and a fine instinct for leisure. . . . He made living a noble gesture.[3]

Should we again remember Frost's noble namesake, Wade Hampton, at Frost's death as we did at his birth? Both men lived lives marked by an "austere sense of duty." Both "made living a noble gesture."

Indeed, Frost's associates did give him the tributes Owens anticipated. Scores of tributes were published in leading medical journals. Among these many, the *American Journal of Public Health and the Nation's Health*, the official publication of the American Public Health Association, commented editorially: "One of the best minds that have adorned the field of public health during this century has passed from us in the untimely death of Wade Hampton Frost."[4]

In 1981, the Department of Epidemiology at Johns Hopkins commissioned a portrait from a photograph (see figure 9.2).

At the dedication of this portrait, Abraham Lilienfeld, who had chaired the department from 1970 to 1975, presented a tribute, the text of which has been framed and hangs near the portrait in the Frost seminar room.

> Epidemiology, as a discipline, provides the underlying scientific foundation for preventive medicine and the practice of public health. Wade Hampton Frost, the first professor and Chairman of the Department of Epidemiology of The Johns Hopkins School of Hygiene and Public Health, played a principal role in the development of epidemiology as an academic discipline and in the recognition of its importance in the practice of public health.
>
> Prior to organizing the first formal academic department of epidemiology in the world, Frost served in the US Public Health Service for fourteen years. He was involved in field work concerned with the control of a yellow fever epidemic, and was later assigned to the Hygienic Laboratory, predecessor of the National Institutes of Health, where he became familiar with the epidemiology and control of such diseases as typhoid fever, septic sore throat, and poliomyelitis. Frost directed the program of research of the pollution of the Ohio River which included chemical, microbiological, and engineering studies. His field investigation of the poliomyelitis epidemic in New York City in 1916 remains an epidemiologic classic.
>
> On assuming the Professorship at Hopkins in 1919, Frost developed the laboratory method of teaching epidemiology in which students dealt with actual data. His studies of diphtheria, the common cold, influenza, and tuberculosis conducted jointly with students and colleagues, led to the use and further development of methods of study and analysis such as life tables, person years, cohort analysis or mortality, and morbidity surveys. Together with Lowell Reed, Professor of Biostatistics, Frost developed the Reed-Frost model for studying the occurrence of epidemics of communicable diseases.
>
> As a teacher, Wade Hampton Frost stressed the need for meticulous care in the collection of data, innovative methods of analysis and critical judgment in deriving inferences. In both research and teaching, he emphasized the integral relationship between epidemiology and the practice of teaching public health.[5]

The American Public Health Association awarded Frost its prestigious Sedgwick Memorial Medal shortly before his death. The citation accompanying this medal read, in part:

> His rigorous honesty of approach and a fine scorn for any other facts than those of enduring worth drew to him students and colleagues who

Table 11.1.

Major contributions of Wade Hampton Frost to the epidemiology of infectious diseases and to epidemiological methods. Adapted, in part, with modifications, from Lilienfeld AM. Wade Hampton Frost: Contributions to epidemiology and public health. *Am J Epidemiol.* **1983; 117:379–83.**

Epidemiology of infectious diseases

- Pathogenesis of poliomyelitis. Understanding the role of asymptomatic childhood infections in spreading infection and producing immunity.
- Cyclical nature of influenza epidemics and utility of tracking outbreaks with excess pneumonia deaths.
- Cyclical occurrence of outbreaks of common colds.
- Immunity to diphtheria toxin in carriers.
- Declining tuberculosis mortality and incidence resulting in a shift of peak rates from young adults to the elderly.

Epidemiological methods

- Index case concept.
- Longitudinal analysis based on age cohorts.
- Use of life tables to express data as person-years.
- Use of life tables to estimate secondary attack rates.
- In collaboration with Lowell Reed, development of a general mathematical expression for the epidemic curve.

cherished the gentle persuasiveness and the judicious encouragement of his helpful criticism. . . . He all but created . . . the scientific discipline and the productive study of epidemiology.[6]

More than a half century has passed since Frost died. Even with this passage of time, Wade Hampton Frost's name stands at the pinnacle of epidemiologists. His major contributions are summarized in table 11.1. Few have taught us more when we have gone to the mountain and walked in their ways.

Bibliography of Publications
by Wade Hampton Frost

1. Anderson JF, Frost WH. The diagnosis of abortive cases of poliomyelitis by the demonstration of specific antibodies. Proceedings of the Society for Experimental Biology and Medicine. 1910; 8:54–56.
2. Frost WH. An organism *(Pseudomonas protea)* isolated from water, agglutinated by the serum of typhoid fever patients. *Hygienic Laboratory Bulletin.* 1910; 66:29–75.
3. Frost WH. Note on an organism isolated from Washington tap water, agglutinated readily by the serum of typhoid fever patients. *American Journal of Pubic Hygiene.* 1910; 20:670–71.
4. Conferences on epidemic poliomyelitis at the meeting of the American Public Health Association, Milwaukee, Wis., September 5–9, 1910. *Public Health Reports.* 1910; 25:1443.
5. Frost WH. The water supply of Williamson, W. Va., and its relation to an epidemic of typhoid fever. *Hygienic Laboratory Bulletin.* 1910; 72:55–90.
6. Frost WH. The field investigation of epidemic poliomyelitis (what the health officer can do toward solving a national problem). *Public Health Reports.* 1910; 25:1663–76.
7. Frost WH. Acute anterior poliomyelitis in New York State in 1910. *Monthly Bulletin of the New York State Department of Health.* 1911; 27:165–184.
8. Anderson JF, Frost WH. Studies upon anaphylaxis with special reference to the antibodies concerned. *Hygienic Laboratory Bulletin.* 1911; 64:1–52.
9. Frost WH. Acute anterior poliomyelitis (infantile paralysis). A précis. *Public Health Bulletin.* 1911; 44:1–52.

10. Anderson JF, Frost WH. Abortive cases of poliomyelitis. An experimental demonstration of specific immune bodies in their blood serum. *Journal of the American Medical Association.* 1911; 56:663–67.

11. Frost WH. Bacteriologic examinations of the water supply. *Hygienic Laboratory Bulletin.* 1911; 78:73–134.

12. Frost WH, Hill HW, Dixon SG. Report of Committee on Methods for the Control of Epidemic Poliomyelitis. *Journal of the American Medical Association.* 1911; 57:1275–78.

13. Frost WH. Origin and prevalence of typhoid fever in Fort Smith, Arkansas, and measures necessary for its control. *Public Health Reports.* 1911; 26:1647–63.

14. Frost WH. Infantile paralysis. Some problems for study by local health officers and practitioners. *Monthly Bulletin of the Ohio State Board of Health.* 1912; 2:79–85.

15. Frost WH. Epidemic cerebrospinal meningitis. A review of its etiology, transmission, and specific therapy, with reference to public measures for its control. *Public Health Reports.* 1912; 27:97–121.

16. Frost WH. Active and passive immunization against plague. *Public Health Reports.* 1912; 27:1361–71.

17. Frost WH. Poliomyelitis. Notes on the discussion at the Fifteenth International Congress on Hygiene and Demography. *Public Health Reports.* 1912; 27:1661–64.

18. Anderson JF, Frost WH. Transmission of poliomyelitis by means of the stable fly (Stomoxys calcitrans). *Public Health Reports.* 1912; 27:1733–35.

19. Frost WH. Septic sore throat: A milk-borne outbreak in Baltimore, MD. Epidemiological study of the outbreak. *Public Health Reports.* 1912; 27:1889–923.

20. Frost WH. Some factors in the epidemiology of poliomyelitis. *American Journal of Public Health.* 1913; 3:216–21.

21. Frost WH. Epidemiologic studies of acute anterior poliomyelitis. I. Poliomyelitis in Iowa, 1910. II. Poliomyelitis in Cincinnati, Ohio, 1911. III. Poliomyelitis in Buffalo and Batavia, N.Y., 1912. *Hygienic Laboratory Bulletin.* 1913; 90:9–252.

22. Frost WH. Conditions contributory to the prevalence of typhoid fever as noted in a sanitary survey of Ohio River cities. *Lancet-Clinic.* 1915; 113:176–79.

23. Frost WH. Some considerations in estimating the sanitary quality of water supplies. *Journal of the American Water Works Association.* 1915; 2:712–34.

24. Frost WH. The activities of the U.S. Public Health Service in epidemiologic studies of infantile paralysis. *Transactions of the American Association for the Study of the Prevention of Infant Mortality.* 1916; 7:180–86.

25. Frost WH. Confirmatory tests for B. coli in routine water examinations. *American Journal of Public Health.* 1916; 6:585–88.

26. Frost WH. Poliomyelitis (infantile paralysis). What is known of its cause and modes of transmission. *Public Health Reports.* 1916; 31:1817–33.

27. Frost WH. The sewage pollution of streams. Its relation to the public health. *Public Health Reports.* 1916; 31:2486–97.

28. Frost WH. Relationship of milk supplies to typhoid fever. *Public Health Reports.* 1916; 31:3291–302.

29. Lavinder CH, Freeman AW, Frost WH. Epidemiologic studies of poliomyelitis in New York City and the Northeastern United States during the year 1916. *Public Health Bulletin.* 1918; 91:1–310.

30. Frost WH, Sydenstricker E. Influenza in Maryland. Preliminary statistics of certain localities. *Public Health Reports.* 1919; 34:491–504.

31. Frost WH, Sydenstricker E. Epidemic influenza in foreign countries. *Public Health Reports.* 1919; 34:1361–76.

32. Frost WH. The epidemiology of influenza. *Public Health Reports.* 1919; 34:1823–36.

33. Frost WH. The epidemiology of influenza. *Journal of the American Medical Association.* 1919; 73:313–18.

34. Frost WH. Statistics of influenza morbidity. With special reference to certain factors in case incidence and case fatality. *Public Health Reports.* 1920; 35:584–97.

35. Frost WH. The development and scope of organized public health endeavor. *Public Health* (Lansing, Michigan). 1922; 10:436–41.

36. Frost WH. Significance of B. coli in water. *Public Health Bulletin.* 1922; 128:47–52.

37. Frost WH. The importance of epidemiology as a function of health departments. *Medical Officer* (London). 1923; 29:113–14.

38. Frost WH. Correlation of sources of pollution. *Engineers and Engineering.* 1923; 15:301–304.

39. Frost WH, Streeter HW. Bacteriolgical studies. *Public Health Bulletin.* 1924; 143:184–341.

40. Frost WH. Rendering account in public health. *American Journal of Public Health.* 1925; 15:394–98.

41. Frost WH. Transactions of the twenty-third annual conference of State and Territorial Health Officers with the United States Public Health Service Held at Washington, D.C. June 1 and 2, 1925. *Public Health Bulletin.* 1926; 161:89, 93–97, 108–109.

42. Frost WH. A review of the work of the United States Public Health Service in investigations of stream pollution. *Transactions of the American Society of Civil Engineers.* 1926; 89:1332–40.

43. Frost WH. A review of the work of the United States Public Health Service in investigations of stream pollution. *Public Health Reports.* 1926; 41:75–85.

44. Frost WH. Transactions of the twenty-fourth annual conference of State and Territorial Health Officers with the United States Public Health Service Held at Washington, D.C. May 24 and 25, 1926. *Public Health Bulletin.* 1927; 167:21–23, 24.

45. Frost WH. Recognition of poliomyelitis. *Ohio Health News.* 1927; 3:1–3.

46. Frost WH. Transactions of the twenty-fifth annual conference of State and Territorial Health Officers with the United States Public Health Service Held at Washington, D.C. May 20 and 21, 1927. *Public Health Bulletin.* 1928; 178:65–66, 68–69.

47. Frost WH. Infection, immunity and disease in the epidemiology of diphtheria. With special reference to some studies in Baltimore. *Journal of Preventive Medicine.* 1928; 2:325–43.

48. Frost WH. Chapter 7. Epidemiology. In Emerson H, ed. *Nelson Loose-Leaf System. Preventive Medicine Public Health.* Vol.2. New York, Thomas Nelson & Sons; 1928: 163–190.

49. Collins SD, Frost WH, Gover M, Sydenstricker E. Mortality from influenza and pneumonia in 50 large cities of the United States, 1910–1929. *Public Health Reports.* 1930; 45:2277–328.

50. Carter HR, Carter LA, Frost WH, eds. *Yellow Fever: An Epidemiological and Historical Study of Its Place of Origin.* Baltimore: Williams & Wilkins; 1931.

51. Wheeler RE, Doull JA, Frost WH. Antitoxic immunity to diphtheria in relation to tonsillectomy. *American Journal of Hygiene.* 1931; 14:555–59.

52. Frost WH, Gover M. The incidence and time distribution of common colds in several groups kept under continuous observation. *Public Health Reports.* 1932; 47:1815–41.

53. Van Volkenburgh VA, Frost WH. Acute minor respiratory diseases prevailing in a group of families residing in Baltimore, Maryland, 1928–1930. Prevalence, distribution and clinical description of observed cases. *American Journal of Hygiene.* 1933; 17:122–53.

54. Frost WH. Risk of persons in familial contact with pulmonary tuberculosis. *American Journal of Public Health and the Nation's Health.* 1933; 23:426–32.

55. Frost WH, Van Volkenburgh VA. The minor respiratory diseases as observed during the influenza epidemic of 1928–29 and in a non-epidemic period. *American Journal of Hygiene.* 1935; 21:647–64.

56. Frost WH. The outlook for the eradication of tuberculosis. *American Review of Tuberculosis.* 1935; 32:644–50.

57. Frost WH. Introduction. *Snow on Cholera. Being a Reprint of Two Papers by John Snow, M.D.* New York: The Commonwealth Fund; 1936.

58. Frost WH. Authoritative standards and Association policy. *American Journal of Public Health and the Nation's Health*, April 1936; 26:336–42.
59. Frost WH, Frobisher M Jr, Van Volkenburgh VA, Levin ML. Diphtheria in Baltimore: A comparative study of morbidity, carrier prevalence and antitoxic immunity in 1921–24 and 1933–36. *American Journal of Hygiene*. 1936; 24:568–86.
60. Frost WH. How much control of tuberculosis? *American Journal of Public Health and the Nation's Health*. 1937; 27:759–66.
61. Frost WH. The familial aggregation of infectious diseases. *American Journal of Public Health*. 1938; 28:7–13.
62. Frost WH. The age selection of mortality from tuberculosis in successive decades. *American Journal of Hygiene*. 1939; 30:91–96.
63. Frost WH. Some conceptions of epidemics in general. *American Journal of Epidemiology*. 1976; 103:141–51.

Abbreviations of Scientific Journal Titles

The titles of scientific journals have been abbreviated in all citations in this work. The abbreviations employed are in conformity with the usage of the National Library of Medicine. A list of these abbreviations with the complete journal names follows.

Am J Epidemiol	American Journal of Epidemiology
Am J Hyg	American Journal of Hygiene
Am J Publ Health	American Journal of Public Health
Am J Publ Health Nations Health	American Journal of Public Health and the Nation's Health
Am J Public Hyg	American Journal of Public Hygiene
Am Rev Respir Dis	American Review of Respiratory Disease
Am Rev Tuberc	American Review of Tuberculosis
Ann Inst Pasteur	Annales de l'Institut Pasteur
Bull Hist Med	Bulletin of the History of Medicine
C R Seances Soc Bio Fil	Comptes Rendus des Séances de la Société de Biologie et de ses Filiales
Hygienic Lab Bull	Hygienic Laboratory Bulletin
Int J Tuberc Lung Dis	International Journal of Tuberculosis and Lung Disease
J Am Med Assoc	Journal of the American Medical Association
J Am Water Works Assoc	Journal of American Water Works Association
J Lab Clin Med	Journal of Laboratory and Clinical Medicine
J Prev Med	Journal of Preventive Medicine
Medical Rec	Medical Record
Microbiol Rev	Microbiological Reviews
Mil Med	Military Medicine
Mon Bull NY State Dep Health	Monthly Bulletin of the New York State Department of Health
Mon Bull Ohio State Board Health	Monthly bulletin of the Ohio State Board of Health
Morbid Mortal Wkly Rep	Morbidity and Mortality Weekly Report
Philos Trans R Soc Lond	Philosophical Transactions of the Royal Society of London
Proc Soc Exp Biol Med	Proceedings of the Society for Experimental Biology and Medicine
Public Health Bull	Public Health Bulletin
Public Health Rep	Public Health Reports
Soz Praventivmed	Sozial und Praventivmedizin
Va Med Q	Virginia Medical Quarterly

Notes

Foreword

1. Frost WH. The age selection of mortality from tuberculosis in successive decades. *Am J Hyg.* 1939; 30:91–96.

2. Paul JR. *Clinical Epidemiology.* Rev. ed. Chicago: The University of Chicago Press; 1966: 30–31.

3. Lilienfeld AM. Epidemiology of infectious and non-infectious disease: The first Wade Hampton Frost lecture. Some comparisons. *AM J Epidemiol.* 1973; 97: 135–47.

4. Fox JP. Family-based epidemiologic studies. The second Wade Hampton Frost lecture. *Am J Epidemiol.* 1974; 99:165–79.

5. Cassel J. The contribution of the social environment to host resistance. The fourth Wade Hampton Frost lecture. *Am J Epidemiol.* 1976; 104:107–23. Frost's statement quoted by Cassel is from Frost WH. Introduction. *Snow on Cholera. Being a Reprint of Two Papers by John Snow, M.D. together with a Biographical Memoir by B.W. Richardson, M.D. and Introduction by Wade Hampton Frost, M.D. Professor of Epidemiology, the Johns Hopkins School of Hygiene and Public health* (Facsimile of 1936 Edition). New York: Hafner Publishing Company; 1965: ix.

6. Terris M. The epidemiologic tradition. The Wade Hampton Frost lecture. *Public Health Rep.* 1979; 94:203–209.

7. Ibid. These last two sentences are ingrained in my memory. The second sentence appears on Mann's monument and is the part quoted by Terris.

8. Comstock GW. Cohort analysis: W.H. Frost's contributions to the epidemiology of tuberculosis and chronic disease. *Soz Praventivmed.* 2001; 46:7–12.

By What Name?

1. Frost WH. Some reasons (editorial). *College Topics.* October 15, 1902.

2. This story of Frost's baptism and naming may be apocryphal. It was repeatedly told within the Frost family and by his daughter, Susan Frost Parrish, to her friends. See also Gwaltney JM Jr. Wade Hampton Frost, MD.: A wider view of the world. *Virginia Med Quarterly.* 1995; 122:261–64.

3. Biographical information on Wade Hampton is available from many sources. A useful biography is provided by Wellman MW. *Giant in Gray: A Biography of Wade Hampton of South Carolina.* New York: Charles Scribner's Sons; 1949.

4. Cauthen CC. *Family Letters of the Three Wade Hamptons 1782–1901.* Columbia, SC: University of South Carolina Press; 1953: 94.

5. Parrish SF. Undated note deposited in the Claude Moore Health Sciences Library, University of Virginia Health Sciences Center, Charlottesville, VA: Wade Hampton Frost Archives, Box 12, Folder 7.

6. The Parish Leaflet, Whittle Parish, Fauquier County, Virginia, May 1917. Claude Moore Health Sciences Library, University of Virginia Health Sciences Center, Charlottesville, VA: Wade Hampton Frost Archives, Box 1, Folder 44.

2: Origins

1. Letter. WH Frost to John T. Ramey, dated November 29, 1895, written from the Danville Military Institute. Claude Moore Health Sciences Library, University of Virginia Health Sciences Center, Charlottesville, VA: Wade Hampton Frost Archives, Box 3, Folder 59.

2. Letter. WH Frost to HC Frost, April 5, 1933. Claude Moore Health Sciences Library, University of Virginia Health Sciences Center, Charlottesville, VA: Wade Hampton Frost Archives, Box 1, Folder 40. Letter, HC Frost to WH Frost, February 8, 1934. Claude Moore Health Sciences Library, University of Virginia Health Sciences Center, Charlottesville, VA: Wade Hampton Frost Archives, Box 1, Folder 41. Pedigree of Thomas Crawshay Frost, Esquire. Claude Moore Health Sciences Library, University of Virginia Health Sciences Center, Charlottesville, VA: Wade Hampton Frost Archives, Box 1, Folder 26.

3. Frost TG, Frost EL. *The Frost Family in America.* Buffalo, NY: Russell Printing Company; 1909. Copies of pages from this book relevant to WH Frost are deposited in the Claude Moore Health Sciences Library, University of Virginia Health Sciences Center, Charlottesville, VA: Wade Hampton Frost Archives, Box 1, Folder 31. These pages contain notes penciled by Susan Haxall Frost (wife of WH Frost) and Susan Frost Parrish (daughter of WH Frost).

4. Ibid. Letter, FR Frost to WH Frost, February 1, 1927. Claude Moore Health Sciences Library, University of Virginia Health Sciences Center, Charlottesville, VA: Wade Hampton Frost Archives, Box 1, Folder 41. Parrish SF. Note dated Feb 1, 1927. Claude Moore Health Sciences Library, University of Virginia Health Sciences Center, Charlottesville, VA: Wade Hampton Frost Archives, Box 11, Folder 18. Stocker AF. Letter dated February 25, 1966 to Frank Berkeley. Claude Moore Health Sciences Library, University of Virginia Health Sciences Center, Charlottesville, VA: Wade Hampton Frost Archives, Box 1, Folder 43.

5. Holcomb BH. *South Carolina Marriages, 1699–1799.* Baltimore, MD: Genealogical Publishing Company, Inc.; 1980: 87. The year of the marriage is incorrectly given in Frost TG, Frost EL. This latter work also gives the wife's last name as Downs, in conflict with other sources that spell it Downes.

6. Ibid.

7. *South Carolina Historical and Genealogical Magazine* 1926; 27:227–28. Claude Moore Health Sciences Library, University of Virginia Health Sciences Center, Charlottesville, VA: Wade Hampton Frost Archives, Box 11, Folder 18.

8. Letter, FR Frost to WH Frost, February 1, 1927. Claude Moore Health Sciences Library, University of Virginia Health Sciences Center, Charlottesville, VA: Wade Hampton Frost Archives, Box 1, Folder 41.

9. Parrish SF. Note dated February 1, 1927. Claude Moore Health Sciences Library, University of Virginia Health Sciences Center, Charlottesville, VA: Wade Hampton Frost Archives, Box 11, Folder 18.

10. Waring JI. *A History of Medicine in South Carolina 1825–1900*. Columbia, SC: South Carolina Medical Association; 1967: 281.

11. Frost TG, Frost EL, op. cit.

12. Hafner AW. *Directory of Deceased American Physicians 1804–1929*. Volume 1. Chicago, IL: American Medical Association; 1993: 538.

13. Apprenticeship, followed by a didactic course in a medical school, and sometimes followed by further hospital experience, was the norm for medical education in the eighteenth and nineteenth centuries. Frost's education closely paralleled that of John Keats, for example; see Daniel TM. *Captain of Death: the Story of Tuberculosis*. Rochester, NY: University of Rochester Press; 1997: 101–103.

14. Waring JI. 1967, op. cit.: 230–32. Parrish SF. Transcript of obituary of Henry R. Frost published in the Charleston Courier, April 9, 1886. Claude Moore Health Sciences Library, University of Virginia Health Sciences Center, Charlottesville, VA: Wade Hampton Frost Archives, Box 12, Folder 01.

15. Waring JI. *A History of Medicine in South Carolina 1670–1825*. Columbia, SC: South Carolina Medical Association; 1964: 160–72. Waring JI, 1967, op. cit. Kelley HA. *A Cyclopedia of American Medical Biography*. Philadelphia, PA: W.B. Saunders Company, 1912.

16. Waring JI, 1967, op. cit.

17. Ibid.

18. Parrish SF. Transcript of obituary of Henry R. Frost published in the *Charleston Courier*, April 9, 1886. Claude Moore Health Sciences Library, University of Virginia Health Sciences Center, Charlottesville, VA: Wade Hampton Frost Archives, Box 12, Folder 01.

19. Ibid.

20. Parrish SF. Hand-written marginal note on transcript of obituary of Henry R. Frost published in the *Charleston Courier*, April 9, 1886. Claude Moore Health Sciences Library, University of Virginia Health Sciences Center, Charlottesville, VA: Wade Hampton Frost Archives, Box 12, Folder 01.

21. Landrum JBO. *History of Spartanburg County*. Atlanta, GA: The Franklin Printing and Publishing Company; 1900: 86–90. Brasington JM. *The South Carolina School for the Deaf and Blind*. Spartanburg, SC: South Carolina School for the Deaf and Blind; 2000. Memorial Edition—Newton Farmer Walker. *The Palmetto Leaf*, February 26, 1927. Deposited in the Claude Moore Health Sciences Library, University of Virginia Health Sciences Center, Charlottesville, VA: Wade Hampton Frost Archives, Box 12, Folder 8. Valuable Service Performed by State School for Deaf and Blind. Undated and unidentified newspaper clipping deposited by Susan Frost Parrish in the Claude Moore Health Sciences Library, University of Virginia Health Sciences Center, Charlottesville, VA: Wade Hampton Frost Archives, Box 11, Folder 16. The information available from these sources is limited. My search of other standard genealogical sources has been fruitless, partly because many individuals named Walker lived in the Spartanburg area, but the names of

Newton Pinckney Walker's parents are unknown. Efforts by Frost to trace this part of his ancestry were nonproductive, as were similar efforts made by Susan Frost Parrish.

22. The chronology of the post-Civil War events of the Frost family has been difficult to reconstruct, and there are few documents or records upon which one can rely. Those available sometimes give conflicting or inconsistent dates. The account here is based on the author's best judgement in interpreting accounts given in Frost TG, Frost EL. Op. cit; Hafner AW., op. cit; *The Parish Leaflet*. Whittle Parish, Fauquier County, Virginia, May 1917. Claude Moore Health Sciences Library, University of Virginia Health Sciences Center, Charlottesville, VA: Wade Hampton Frost Archives, Box 1, Folder 44; and Brasington JM., op. cit.

23. Ayers EL, Willis JC, eds. *The Edge of the South: Life in Nineteenth-Century Virginia*. Charlottesville, VA: University Press of Virginia; 1991.

24. Cunningham, MR. Interview with the author, August 23, 2001.

3: Marshall

1. Letter, WH Frost to J Ramey, November 29, 1895. Claude Moore Health Sciences Library, University of Virginia Health Sciences Center, Charlottesville, VA: Wade Hampton Frost Archives, Box 3, Folder 59.

2. Gott JK. *High in Old Virginia's Piedmont: A History of Marshall (Formerly Salem), Fauquier County, Virginia*. Marshall, VA: Marshall National Bank and Trust Company; 1987. Gott JK. Interview with the author, 2001. Cunningham M. Interview with the author, 2001. Gott's book is a useful history of Marshall; the interviews with Gott and long-time resident, Mary Cunningham, provided many additional details included in the descriptions of Marshall in this chapter.

3. Groome HC. *Fauquier During the Proprietorship: A Chronicle of the Colonization of a Northern Neck "County*. Baltimore, MD: Regional Publishing Company; 1969. Anonymous. *Fauquier County, Virginia, 1759–1959*. Warrenton, VA: Fauquier County Bicentennial Committee; 1959.

4. Gott JK, 2001, op. cit.

5. Gott JK. 1987, op. cit. Hammant MF. Old Salem (now Marshall) as it was in the Old Days. *Fauquier Democrat*, May 10, 1956.

6. *The Parish Leaflet*. Whittle Parish, Fauquier County, Virginia, May 1917. Claude Moore Health Sciences Library, University of Virginia Health Sciences Center, Charlottesville, VA: Wade Hampton Frost Archives, Box 1, Folder 44.

7. Gott JK, 2001, op. cit.

8. Statement rendered to John Glascock by Henry Frost, M.D. December 1, 1903. Archives of the Fauquier County Heritage Society, Marshall, VA.

9. Ten great public health achievements—United States, 1900–1999. *Morbid Mortal Wkly Rep*. 1999; 48:241–48. Achievements in public health, 1900–1999. Control of infectious diseases. *Morbid Mortal Wkly Rep*. 1999; 48:621–29.

10. Blanton WB. *Medicine in Virginia in the Nineteenth Century*. Richmond, VA: Garrett & Massie, Incorporated; 1933:98.

11. Williams RC. *The United States Public Health Service, 1798–1950*. Washington, DC: Commissioned Officers Association of the United States Public Health Service; 1951: 61.

12. Frost TG, Frost EL. *The Frost Family in England and America with Special Reference to Edmund Frost and Some of his Descendants*. Buffalo, NY. Russell Printing Company; 1909. Claude Moore Health Sciences Library, University of Virginia Health Sciences Center, Charlottesville, VA: Wade Hampton Frost Archives, Box 1, Folder 31.

13. Parrish SF. Undated note. Claude Moore Health Sciences Library, University of Virginia Health Sciences Center, Charlottesville, VA: Wade Hampton Frost Archives, Box 81, Folder 12.

14. *The Parish Leaflet*, 1917, op. cit.

15. H Frost to WH Frost, letter dated July 31, 1913. Claude Moore Health Sciences Library, University of Virginia Health Sciences Center, Charlottesville, VA: Wade Hampton Frost Archives, Box 3, Folder 43.

16. The letters referred to are all at the Claude Moore Health Sciences Library, University of Virginia Health Sciences Center, Charlottesville, VA: Wade Hampton Frost Archives. All are in separate folders of Box 3.

17. Parrish SF. Undated handwritten note. Claude Moore Health Sciences Library, University of Virginia Health Sciences Center, Charlottesville, VA: Wade Hampton Frost Archives, Box 4, Folder 28.

18. Maxcy KF. *Papers of Wade Hampton Frost, M.D.: A Contribution to Epidemiological Method*. New York, NY: The Commonwealth Fund; 1941.

19. Ramey JT. A tribute to my old friend—Wade Frost. *Fauquier Democrat*, May 1938. The precise publication date is unknown. Archived copies of this local newspaper were destroyed in the 1940s. Susan Frost Parish placed this clipping in the Claude Moore Health Sciences Library, University of Virginia Health Sciences Center, Charlottesville, VA: Wade Hampton Frost Archives, Box 4, Folder 28.

20. Cunningham MF, 2001, op. cit.

21. Ibid.

22. Gott JK, 2001, op. cit.

23. Cunningham MR, Turner MF. *1849–1949: A History of Trinity Church, Marshall, Virginia*. Marshall, VA: The Women's Auxillary, Trinity Church; 1949.

24. Gott JK, 2001, op. cit.

25. Ramey JT, 1938, op. cit.

26. Letter, WH Frost to Mrs. Ramey, November 10, 1895. Claude Moore Health Sciences Library, University of Virginia Health Sciences Center, Charlottesville, VA: Wade Hampton Frost Archives, Box 3, Folder 58.

27. Ibid.

28. Frost WH, 1895a, op. cit.

29. Ibid.

30. Ibid.

31. Ibid.

4: Health of the People

1. Frost WH. What every health officer should know. Epidemiology. Typescript. Address prepared for delivery before the 1937 Annual Meeting of the American

Public Health Association. Claude Moore Health Sciences Library, University of Virginia Health Sciences Center, Charlottesville, VA: Wade Hampton Frost Archives, Box 4, Folder 13.

2. Culbreth DMR. *The University of Virginia: Memories of Her Student-Life and Professors*. New York, NY: The Neale Publishing Company; 1908.

3. Patton JS, Doswell SJ. *The University of Virginia: Glimpses of its Past and Present*. Lynchburg, VA: J.P. Bell Company; 1900.

4. Culbreth DMR, op. cit.

5. Information from University of Virginia catalogues kindly provided by Jeanne C. Pardee, Albert and Shirley Small Special Collections Library, University of Virginia.

6. Make up your mind (editorial). *College Topics*, October 8, 1902.

7. Ibid.

8. The martyrdom of Miles (editorial). *College Topics*, October 25, 1902.

9. Crenshaw LD, ed. *A History of the Quinquennial Reunion of the Class of 1908*. Claude Moore Health Sciences Library, University of Virginia Health Sciences Center, Charlottesville, VA: Wade Hampton Frost Archives, Box 11, Folder 11. This reunion booklet was published on the occasion of the fifth reunion of the class of 1908, which was not Frost's class. Frost is clearly identified as the author of these lyrics, and one must presume he wrote them while an undergraduate and that they became sufficiently popular to be in use at least in 1908, five years after he graduated, and perhaps in 1913, when the reunion took place.

10. Heaton CE. *A Historical Sketch of New York University College of Medicine 1841–1941*. New York, NY: New York University; 1941.

11. Daniel TM. *Pioneers of Medicine and Their Impact on Tuberculosis*. Rochester, NY. University of Rochester Press; 2000: 98–131.

12. Maxcy KF. *Papers of Wade Hampton Frost, M.D.: A Contribution to the Epidemiological Method*. New York, NY: The Commonwealth Fund; 1941. Maxcy's major source for the biographical information included in this work was Frost's sister, Harriet Frost. See Parrish SF. Undated handwritten note. Claude Moore Health Sciences Library, University of Virginia Health Sciences Center, Charlottesville, VA: Wade Hampton Frost Archives, Box 4, Folder 28.

13. Maxcy KF, op. cit.

14. Gwaltney JM. Wade Hampton Frost, MD. A Wider View of the World. *Va Med Q*. 1995; 122:261–64.

15. Parrish SF. Transcript of interview by E Fee, May 5, 1982. Claude Moore Health Sciences Library, University of Virginia Health Sciences Center, Charlottesville, VA: Wade Hampton Frost Archives, Box 14, Folder 17.

16. *Corks and Curls*. Volume 16, 1903.

17. Daniel TM, 2000, op. cit.

18. Williams RC. *The United States Public Health Service 1798–1950*. Washington, DC: Commissioned Officers Association of the United States Public Health Service; 1951.

19. Sartwell P. Interview with B Rutizer, June 25, 1975. Claude Moore Health Sciences Library, University of Virginia Health Sciences Center, Charlottesville, VA: Wade Hampton Frost Archives, Box 16, Tape 8.

20. Anderson EB. Interview with B Rutizer, July 23, 1975. Claude Moore Health Sciences Library, University of Virginia Health Sciences Center, Charlottesville, VA: Wade Hampton Frost Archives, Box 16, Tapes 5 and 17.

21. *Public Health Rep.* 1906; 20:1505. The subsequent pages of this volume contain weekly reports detailing the day-by-day course of this outbreak. They have been used as the source for the data and description of this epidemic.

22. McNeill WH. *Plagues and Peoples.* New York, NY: Doubleday; 1977. Clarke DH, Casals J. Arboviruses; Group B. In Horsfall FL, Tamm I., eds. *Viral and Rickettsial Infections of Man.* 4th ed. Philadelphia, PA: J.B. Lippincott Company; 1965: 606–58. Monath TP. Yellow Fever. In Warren KS, Mahmoud AAF, eds. *Tropical and Geographical Medicine.* 2nd ed. New York: McGraw-Hill Information Services; 1990: 661–74.

23. Humphreys M. *Yellow Fever and the South.* New Brunswick, NJ: Rutgers University Press; 1992: 34–38.

24. Bowen TE. William Crawford Gorgas, physician to the world. *Mil Med.* 1983; 148:917–20. Craddock WL. The achievements of William Crawford Gorgas. *Mil Med,* 1997; 162:325–27.

25. *Public Health Rep.* 1906; 20:1510.

26. Ibid: 1507.

27. Ibid: 1622–23.

28. Ibid: 2447.

29. Parrish SF. Notes dated September and November 1984 and deposited with accompanying photographs in Claude Moore Health Sciences Library, University of Virginia Health Sciences Center, Charlottesville, VA: Wade Hampton Frost Archives, Box 6, Folder 18. See also Maxcy KF, op. cit.

30. Parrish SF, 1984, op. cit.

5: Drink No Longer Water

1. Frost WH. Epidemiology. In Havens E, ed. *Nelson Loose-Leaf System: Preventive Medicine and Public Health.* New York, NY: Thomas Nelson & Sons; 1928.

2. 1 Tim. 5:23. Authorized King James version.

3. Duffy J. *The Sanitarians: A History of American Public Health.* Chicago, IL: University of Illinois Press; 1990: 193–204.

4. Frascatorius, Hieronymus Veronensis. The Theory of Infection. In Major RH. *Classic Descriptions of Disease: With Biographical Sketches of the Authors.* 3rd ed. Springfield, IL: Charles C Thomas; 1945: 8.

5. Van Leeuwenhoek A. Microscopical observations about animals in the scurf of the teeth. *Phil Trans R Soc Lond.* 1684; 14:568–74.

6. Doetsch RN. Benjamin Marten and his "New Theory of Consumptions." *Microbiol Rev.* 1978; 42:521–28.

7. For further discussion of the emergence of concepts of infectious diseases see Daniel TM. *Pioneers of Medicine and Their Impact on Tuberculosis.* Chapter 1. Rochester, NY: University of Rochester Press; 2000. See also Daniel TM, Baum GL. *Drama and Discovery: The Story of Histoplasmosis.* Chapter 2. Westport, CT: Greenwood Press; 2002.

8. Daniel TM, 2000, op. cit.

9. H Frost to WH Frost, letter dated July 31, 1913. Claude Moore Health Sciences Library, University of Virginia Health Sciences Center, Charlottesville, VA: Wade Hampton Frost Archives, Box 3, Folder 43.

10. Budd W. *Typhoid Fever: Its Nature, Mode of Spreading, and Prevention.* New York, NY: George Grady Press; 1931. Originally published in London in 1874.

11. Anonymous. Outbreak of fever at the Clergy Orphan School in St. John's Wood. *Lancet.* 1856; 2:555. Budd W. On the fever at the Clergy Orphan Asylum. *Lancet.* 1856; 2:617–19.

12. Budd W, 1931, op. cit.

13. Ibid.

14. Snow J. *On the Mode of Communication of Cholera.* London: John Churchill; 1855. This work was republished in 1936, with an introduction by Wade Hampton Frost, by the Harvard University Press, Cambridge, MA, and again in 1965 by Hafner Publishing Company, New York.

15. Beagle FD. Health legislation. *Twenty-Sixth Annual Report of the State Department of Health of New York.* Vol. 3. Albany: J.B. Lyon Company, 1916:139–48. Williams RC. *The United States Public Health Service, 1798–1950.* Washington, DC: Commissioned Officers Association of the United States Public Health Service, 1951.

16. Achievements in public health, 1900–1999. Control of infectious diseases. *Morbid Mortal Wkly Rep.* 1999; 48:621–29.

17. Daniel, TM, 2000, op. cit: 98–131.

18. Williams RC, op. cit.

19. Frost WH. A review of the work of the United States Public Health Service in investigations of stream pollution. *Public Health Rep.* 1926; 41:75–85.

20. Bureau of the Census. *Mortality Statistics 1908: Ninth Annual Report.* Washington, DC: Government Printing Office; 1910.

21. Stebbins E. Interview with Rutizer B, 1975. Claude Moore Health Sciences Library, University of Virginia Health Sciences Center, Charlottesville, VA: Wade Hampton Frost Archives, Box 16, Tapes 009 and 011.

22. Organization of Hygienic Laboratory. *Hygienic Lab Bull.* 1909; 47:3.

23. Rosenau MJ, Lumsden LL, Kastle JH. Report on the origin and prevalence of typhoid fever in the District of Columbia. *Hygienic Lab Bull.* 1907; 35:1–361. Rosenau MJ, Lumsden LL, Kastle JH. Report No. 2 on the origin and prevalence of typhoid fever in the District of Columbia (1907). *Hygienic Lab Bull.* 1908; 44:1–64. Rosenau MJ, Lumsden LL, Kastle JH. Report No. 3 on the origin and prevalence of typhoid fever in the District of Columbia (1908). *Hygienic Lab Bull.* 1909; 52: 1–162.

24. Stebbins E, 1975, op. cit.

25. Frost WH. Note on an organism from Washington tap water, agglutinated readily by the serum of typhoid fever patients. *Am J Public Hyg.* 1910; 20: 670–71.

26. Frost WH. An organism (*pseudomonas protea*) isolated from water, agglutinated by the serum of typhoid fever patients. *Hygienic Lab Bull.* 1910; 66: 29–75.

27. Frost WH. Bacteriologic examinations of the water supply. *Hygienic Lab Bull.* 1911; 78:73–134.

28. Frost WH. The water supply of Williamson, West Virginia, and its relation to an epidemic of typhoid fever. *Hygienic Lab Bull.* 1910; 72:55–90. Reprinted in

Maxcy KF. *Papers of Wade Hampton Frost, M.D: A contribution to the epidemiological method.* New York, NY: The Commonwealth Fund; 1941: 26–69.

29. Ibid.

30. Ibid.

31. Frost WH. Some considerations in estimating the sanitary quality of water supplies. *J Am Water Works Assoc.* 1915; 2:712–34.

32. Frost WH. Origin and prevalence of typhoid fever in Fort Smith, Ark., and measures necessary for its control. *Public Health Rep.* 1911; 26:1647–63.

33. Ibid.

34. Frost WH. Relationship of milk supplies to typhoid fever. *Public Health Rep.* 1916; 31:3291–302.

35. Anderson JF, Frost WH. Studies upon anaphylaxis with special reference to the antibodies concerned. *Hygienic Lab Bull.* 1910; 64:1–52.

36. Daniel TM, Robbins FC, eds. *Polio.* Rochester, NY: University of Rochester Press; 1997.

37. Netter A, Levaditi C. Action microbicide exercée sur le virus do la poliomyélite aigue par le sérum des sujets antérieurement atteints de paralysie infantiles. Sa contation dans le sérum d'un sujet qui a présenté une forme abortive. *C R Soc Biol Fil.* 1910; 68:855–57.

38. Anderson JF, Frost WH. The diagnosis of abortive cases of poliomyelitis by the demonstration of specific antibodies. *Proc Soc Exp Biol Med.* 1910; 8:54–56. Anderson JF, Frost WH. Abortive cases of poliomyelitis. An experimental demonstration of specific immune bodies in their blood-serum. *J Am Med Assoc.* 1911; 56:663–67.

39. Frost WH. Conferences on epidemic poliomyelitis at the meeting of the American Public Health Association, Milwaukee, Wis., September 5–9, 1910. *Public Health Rep.* 1910; 25:1443.

40. Anderson JF, Frost WH. Transmission of poliomyelitis by means of the stable fly (*Stomoxys calcitrans*). *Public Health Rep.* 1912; 27:1733–35.

41. Sartwell PE. The contributions of Wade Hampton Frost. *Am J Epidemiol.* 1976; 104:386–91.

42. Frost WH. The field investigation of epidemic poliomyelitis (What the public health officer can do toward solving a national problem). *Public Health Rep.* 1910; 25:1663–76.

43. Frost WH. Epidemiologic studies of acute anterior poliomyelitis. I. Poliomyelitis in Iowa, 1910. Poliomyelitis in Cincinnati, Ohio, 1911. Poliomyelitis in Buffalo and Batavia, N.Y., 1912. *Hygienic Lab Bull.* 1913; 90:9–252.

44. Paul JR. *A History of Poliomyelitis.* New Haven, CT: Yale University Press; 1971: 143.

45. Ibid:131–32.

46. Frost WH, 1913, op. cit: 250–51.

47. Frost WH. Acute anterior poliomyelitis in New York State in 1910. *Mon Bull NY State Dep Health.* 1911; 27:165–84.

48. Frost WH. Acute anterior poliomyelitis (infantile paralysis). *Public Health Bull.* 1911; 44:5–53.

49. Frost WH, Hill HW, Dixon SG. Report of committee on methods for the control of epidemic poliomyelitis. *J Am Med Assoc.* 1911; 57:1275–78.

50. Ibid.

51. Frost WH. Infantile paralysis. Some problems for study by local health officers and practitioners. *Mon Bull Ohio State Board Health*. 1912; 79–85. Frost WH. Poliomyelitis. Notes of the discussion at the fifteenth international congress on hygiene and demography. *Public Health Rep*. 1912; 27:1661–64. Frost WH. Some factors in the epidemiology of poliomyelitis. *Am J Public Health Nations Health*. 1913; 3:216–21.

52. Paul JR, 1971, op. cit: 146.

53. Frost WH. Epidemic cerebrospinal meningitis. A review of its etiology, transmission, and specific therapy, with reference to public measures for its control. *Public Health Rep*. 1912; 27: 97–121.

54. Frost WH. Septic sore throat. A milk-borne outbreak in Baltimore, MD. Epidemiological study of the outbreak. *Public Health Rep*. 1912; 27:1889–923.

55. Stebbins E, 1975, op. cit.

56. Frost WH, 1912a, op. cit. Frost WH. Active and passive immunization against plague. *Public Health Rep*. 1912; 27: 1361–71.

6: Susan

1. Frost WH. Introduction. *Snow on Cholera. Being a Reprint of Two Papers by John Snow, M.D. together with a Biographical Memoir by B. W. Richardson, M.D. and an Introduction by Wade Hampton Frost, M.D. Professor of Epidemiology, the Johns Hopkins School of Hygiene and Public Health* (Facsimile of 1936 Edition). New York, NY: Hafner Publishing Company; 1965: xvii.

2. Doull JA. The Bacteriological Era. In Winslow C-EA. *The History of American Epidemiology*. St. Louis, MO: C.V. Mosby Company; 1952: 74–113.

3. Parrish SF. Memorandum to B Rutizer. July 22, 1975. Claude Moore Health Sciences Library, University of Virginia Health Sciences Center, Charlottesville, VA: Wade Hampton Frost Archives, Box 8, Folder 12. Parrish SF. Transcript of interview by Fee E, May 5, 1982. Claude Moore Health Sciences Library, University of Virginia Health Sciences Center, Charlottesville, VA: Wade Hampton Frost Archives, Box 14, Folder 17.

4. Haxall genealogy chart deposited by Susan Frost Parrish in the Claude Moore Health Sciences Library, University of Virginia Health Sciences Center, Charlottesville, VA: Wade Hampton Frost Archives, Box 1, Folder 50. Noland genealogy chart provided by John K. Gott, Fauquier Heritage Society, Marshall, VA. Tyler LG. *Encyclopedia of Virginia Biography*. Vol. 2. New York, NY: Lewis Historical Publishing Company; 1915: 331. Parrish SF. Handwritten note dated November 27, 1975. Claude Moore Health Sciences Library, University of Virginia Health Sciences Center, Charlottesville, VA: Wade Hampton Frost Archives, Box 8, Folder 6. Parrish SF. Handwritten note dated September 1984. Claude Moore Health Sciences Library, University of Virginia Health Sciences Center, Charlottesville, VA: Wade Hampton Frost Archives, Box 1, Folder 47.

5. Parrish SF, 1982, op. cit.

6. Parrish SF. Remarks made during an interview with Mrs. Ivan Marty recorded by B Rutizer. July 23, 1975. Claude Moore Health Sciences Library, University of Virginia Health Sciences Center, Charlottesville, VA: Wade Hampton Frost Archives, Box 16, Tape 6.

7. Parrish SF. Undated typewritten note. Claude Moore Health Sciences Library, University of Virginia Health Sciences Center, Charlottesville, VA: Wade Hampton Frost Archives, Box 7, Folder 32.

8. Parrish SF. Undated notes. Claude Moore Health Sciences Library, University of Virginia Health Sciences Center, Charlottesville, VA: Wade Hampton Frost Archives, Box 8, Folder 20.

9. Parrish SF. 1982, op. cit.

10. Cunningham M. Interview with the author, 2001.

11. The death certificate gave the cause of death as cholera. While cholera was common in ocean port cities where it was imported by ships carrying immigrants, reliable laboratory means for its diagnosis were not yet available. Hence, it is difficult to be sure that the child's illness was indeed cholera. However, if it was some other diarrheal disease, the public health implications are the same, for sewage-polluted water was a major cause of diarrheal disease at that time.

12. Frost WH. The sewage pollution of streams: Its relation to he public health. *Public Health Rep.* 1916; 31:2486–97. Reprinted in Maxcy KF. *Papers of Wade Hampton Frost, M.D. A Contribution to the Epidemiologic Method.* New York, NY: The Commonwealth Fund; 1941: 287–301.

13. Williams RC. *The United States Public Health Service 1798–1950.* Washington, DC: Commissioned Officers of the United States Public Health Service; 1951:312–16. Furman B. *A Profile of the United States Public Health Service 1798–1948.* Washington, DC: U.S. Department of Health, Education and Welfare, National Institutes of Health, National Library of Medicine; 1973. DHEW Publication No. (NIH) 73–369:294–98.

14. Department of Commerce. Bureau of the Census. *Mortality Statistics 1913: Fourteenth Annual Report.* Washington, DC: Government Printing Office; 1915.

15. Frost WH. Conditions contributory to the prevalence of typhoid fever as noted in a sanitary survey of Ohio River cities. *Lancet-Clinic.* 1915; 113: 176–79.

16. Ibid.

17. Wolman A. Interview recorded by B Rutizer. June 26, 1975. Claude Moore Health Sciences Library, University of Virginia Health Sciences Center, Charlottesville, VA: Wade Hampton Frost Archives, Box 16, Tape 24.

18. Frost WH. Some considerations in estimating the sanitary quality of water supplies. *J Am Water Works Assoc.* 1915; 2:712–22. Reprinted in Maxcy KF, op. cit. Quoted with permission. Copyright 1915. American Water Works Association.

19. Ibid.

20. Frost WH. A review of the work of the United States Public Health Service in investigations of stream pollution. *Public Health Rep.* 1926; 41:75–85. Reprinted in Maxcy KF, op. cit.

21. WT Sedgwick to S Haxall, December 26, 1914. Claude Moore Health Sciences Library, University of Virginia Health Sciences Center, Charlottesville, VA: Wade Hampton Frost Archives, Box 2, Folder 53.

22. WT Sedgwick to WH Frost, December 27, 1914. Claude Moore Health Sciences Library, University of Virginia Health Sciences Center, Charlottesville, VA: Wade Hampton Frost Archives, Box 2, Folder 52.

23. H Frost to WH Frost, January 21, 1915. Claude Moore Health Sciences Library, University of Virginia Health Sciences Center, Charlottesville, VA: Wade Hampton Frost Archives, Box 3, Folder 45.

24. WT Sedgwick to WH Frost, December 27, 1914, op. cit.

25. Parrish SF. Note dated August 24, 1985. Claude Moore Health Sciences Library, University of Virginia Health Sciences Center, Charlottesville, VA: Wade Hampton Frost Archives, Box 9, Folder 42.

26. Frost H. Letters to WH Frost, 1915–1916. Claude Moore Health Sciences Library, University of Virginia Health Sciences Center, Charlottesville, VA: Wade Hampton Frost Archives, Box 3, Folders 46–50.

27. Anderson EB. Interview recorded by B Rutizer, July 23, 1975. Claude Moore Health Sciences Library, University of Virginia Health Sciences Center, Charlottesville, VA: Wade Hampton Frost Archives, Box 16, Tape 17.

28. Frost WH, 1915a, op. cit.

29. WH Frost to C.B. Cook, November 16, 1914. Claude Moore Health Sciences Library, University of Virginia Health Sciences Center, Charlottesville, VA: Wade Hampton Frost Archives, Box 15, Folder 3.

30. R Blue to J Marshall, January 26, 1915. Claude Moore Health Sciences Library, University of Virginia Health Sciences Center, Charlottesville, VA: Wade Hampton Frost Archives, Box 15, Folder 3. The complete correspondence regarding this incident can be found in this archive folder.

31. Frost WH, 1915a, op. cit. Frost WH. The sewage pollution of streams. Its relation to the public health. *Public Health Rep.* 1916; 31:2486–97.

32. Paul JR. *A History of Poliomyelitis.* New Haven, CT: Yale University Press; 1971: 148–60.

33. Daniel TM, Robbins FC, eds. *Polio.* Rochester, NY: University of Rochester Press; 1997.

34. Daniel TM. *Pioneers of Medicine and their Impact on Tuberculosis.* Rochester, NY: University of Rochester Press; 2000: 96–131.

35. A brief account of the New York City epidemic is given by Paul JR, 1971, op. Cit. For a more detailed account, see Lavinder CH, Freeman AW, Frost WH. Epidemiologic studies of poliomyelitis in New York City and the northeastern United States during the year 1916. *Public Health Bull.* 1918; 91:1–310.

36. Williams, RC, 1951, op. cit: 204.

37. H Frost to WH Frost, October 2, 1916. Claude Moore Health Sciences Library, University of Virginia Health Sciences Center, Charlottesville, VA: Wade Hampton Frost Archives, Box 3, Folder 51.

38. Lavinder CH, Freeman AW, Frost WH, 1918, op. cit. See also Paul JR, 1971, op. cit.

39. Lavinder CH, Freeman AW, Frost WH, 1918, op. cit.

40. Frost WH. Poliomyelitis (infantile paralysis). What is known of its cause and modes of transmission. *Public Health Rep.* 1916; 31:1817–33.

41. Frost WH, 1926, op. cit.

42. Transactions of the twenty-third annual conference of state and territorial health officers of the United States Public Health Service. *Public Health Bull.* 1926;

161:89–113. Transactions of the twenty-fourth annual conference of state and territorial health officers of the United States Public Health Service. *Public Health Bull.* 1927; 167:21–26. Transactions of the twenty-fifth annual conference of state and territorial health officers of the United States Public Health Service. *Public Health Bull.* 1928; 178:65–68.

    43. Maxcy KF, op. cit: 9.

7: Dread Diseases

    1. Frost WH. Epidemiology. In Emerson H, ed. *Nelson Loose-Leaf System: Preventive Medicine and Public Health*. New York, NY: Thomas Nelson & Sons; 1928.

    2. Dickens C. *Nicholas Nickleby*. London: Penguin Books; 1986: 731. Originally published in 1839. Although Dickens did not specifically state that the wasting disease that afflicted Nicholas's friend, Smike, was tuberculosis, the context of the story leaves little doubt that it was.

    3. Furman B. *A Profile of the United States Public health Service 1978–1948*. Washington, DC: U.S. Department of Health Education and Welfare, National Institutes of Health, national Library of Medicine; 1973. DHEW Publication No. (NIH) 73–369: 314.

    4. Frost WH. Undated draft of a memorandum entitled General Understanding of Public Health in the Civil Population During the War. Claude Moore Health Sciences Library, University of Virginia Health Sciences Center, Charlottesville, VA: Wade Hampton Frost Archives, Box 11, Folder 29.

    5. Daniel TM. *Captain of Death: The Story of Tuberculosis*. Rochester, NY: University of Rochester Press; 1997.

    6. Grigg ERN. The arcana of tuberculosis with a brief history of the disease in the U.S.A. *Am Rev Tuberc.* 1958; 78:151–72, 426–53, 583–603.

    7. Centers for Disease control and Prevention. Reported Tuberculosis in the United States, 2003. Atlanta, GA, 2002.

    8. Daniel, 1997, op. cit. For an elegant description of the early sanatorium movement, see also Davis AL. History of the Sanatorium Movement. In Rom WN, Garay SM, eds. *Tuberculosis*. New York, NY: Little, Brown and Company; 1996. Also, Rothman SM. *Living in the Shadow of Death: Tuberculosis and the Social Experience of Illness in American History*. New York, NY: Basic Books; 1994.

    9. Knopf SA. *A History of the National Tuberculosis Association: The Anti-Tuberculosis Movement in the United States*. New York, NY: National Tuberculosis Association; 1922: 376–78. Knopf gives the date of Minor's tuberculosis and move to Asheville as 1884, but this date is clearly in error. The correct date is probably 1894.

    10. WT Sedgwick to WH Frost, November 16, 1917. Claude Moore Health Sciences Library, University of Virginia Health Sciences Center, Charlottesville, VA: Wade Hampton Frost Archives, Box 9, Folder 42. As noted earlier in the text, Sedgwick was a sanitary engineer on the faculty of the Massachusetts Institute of Technology. He served as a member of the Advisory Board of the Hygienic

Laboratory of the Public Health Service while Frost was stationed there and working on stream pollution.

11. WT Sedgwick to WH Frost, November 16, 1917. Claude Moore Health Sciences Library, University of Virginia Health Sciences Center, Charlottesville, VA: Wade Hampton Frost Archives, Box 9, Folder 42. The American Clinical and Climatological Association was, at that time, an elite professional society of physicians devoted to the care of patients with tuberculosis and research upon that disease. It drew its name from the then current belief in the beneficial effects of certain climates and of what was often termed "the outdoor life."

12. Mann T. *The Magic Mountain.* New York, NY: Vintage Books; 1992: 182.

13. Minor C, op. cit.

14. Maxcy KF, ed. *Papers of Wade Hampton Frost, M.D.: A Contribution to the Epidemiological Method.* New York, NY: The Commonwealth Fund; 1941.

15. Sartwell PE. Interview recorded by B Rutizer in 1975. Claude Moore Health Sciences Library, University of Virginia Health Sciences Center, Charlottesville, VA: Wade Hampton Frost Archives, Box 16, Tape 8.

16. Zeidberg LD, Gass RS, Dillon A, Hutcheson RH. The Williamson County tuberculosis study. A twenty-four-year epidemiologic study. *Am Rev Respir Dis.* 1963; 87(Suppl):1–88.

17. Mann T, op. cit: 327.

18. CL Minor to SH Frost, April 29, 1918. Claude Moore Health Sciences Library, University of Virginia Health Sciences Center, Charlottesville, VA: Wade Hampton Frost Archives, Box 9, Folder 34.

19. Alling DW, Bosworth EB. The after-history of pulmonary tuberculosis. VI. The first fifteen years following diagnosis. *Am Rev Respir Dis.* 1960; 81:839–49.

20. Daniel Tm, Baum GL. *Drama and Discovery: The Story of Histoplasmosis.* Westport, CT: Greenwood Press; 2002.

21. Daniel TM, 1997, op. cit: 104.

22. Trudeau EL. *An Autobiography.* Philadelphia, PA: Lea & Febiger; 1915: 71.

23. Anderson EB. Interview recorded by B Rutiser in 1975. Claude Moore Health Sciences Library, University of Virginia Health Sciences Center, Charlottesville, VA: Wade Hampton Frost Archives, Box 16, Tape 17. This interview is the only existing documentation of Henry Pickney Frost's illness; the disease of Thomas Lownes Frost is well documented in many sources.

24. WH Frost to TL Frost, May 8, 1922. Claude Moore Health Sciences Library, University of Virginia Health Sciences Center, Charlottesville, VA: Wade Hampton Frost Archives, Box 3, Folder 84. Frost's use of the word "sanitarium" in place of "sanatorium" is interesting. Although the two words have often been used interchangeably, sanitarium more commonly meant a spa rather than a tuberculosis hospital, which the latter word designated. One can suppose that Frost's usage was accidental, but Frost was such a man of detail that it seems unlikely.

25. Frost WH. Handwritten fragment of letter to TL Frost dated March 15, 1923. Claude Moore Health Sciences Library, University of Virginia Health Sciences Center, Charlottesville, VA: Wade Hampton Frost Archives, Box 3, Folder 89.

26. Daniel TM. *Pioneers in Medicine and Their Impact on Tuberculosis.* Rochester, NY: University of Rochester Press: 2000: 36–61.

27. Johnson NPAS, Mueller J. Updating the accounts: Global mortality of the 1918–1920 "Spanish" influenza epidemic. *Bull Hist Med.* 2002; 76:105–15.

28. Daniel TM, Gerstner PA. The 1918–1919 influenza pandemic. *J Lab Clin Med.* 1991; 117:259–60. Crosby AW Jr. *Epidemic and Peace, 1918.* Westport, CT: Greenwood Press; 1976. Tuabenberger JK. Seeking the 1918 Spanish influenza virus. *ASM News.* 1999; 65:473–78.

29. Webster RG. A molecular whodunit. *Science.* 2001; 293:1773–75. Gibbs MJ, Armstrong JS, Gibbs AJ. Recombination in the hemagglutinin gene of the 1918 "Spanish flu." *Science.* 2001; 293:1842–45.

30. Daniel TM, Gerstner PA, 1991, op. cit.

31. *Public Health Rep.* 1918; 33:502. Crosby AW Jr, 1976, op. cit: 18.

32. WH Frost to "Surgeon General," April 19, 1919. Claude Moore Health Sciences Library, University of Virginia Health Sciences Center, Charlottesville, VA: Wade Hampton Frost Archives, Box 15, Folder 02.

33. Doull JA. III. The Bacteriological Era (1876–1920). In Top FH, ed. *The History of American Epidemiology.* St. Louis, MO: The C.V. Mosby Company; 1952: 102.

34. *Public Health Rep.* 1918; 33:1729.

35. *Public Health Rep.* 1918; 33:1822.

36. Crosby AW Jr, 1976, op. cit: 205.

37. Frost WH. Report of Progress in Statistical and Epidemiological Studies of Influenza During Fiscal Year Ending June 30, 1919. Typescript deposited in the Claude Moore Health Sciences Library, University of Virginia Health Sciences Center, Charlottesville, VA: Wade Hampton Frost Archives, Box 15, Folder 02.

38. Frost WH, Sydenstricker E. Epidemic influenza in foreign countries. *Public Health Rep.* 1919; 34:1361–76.

39. Frost WH. The epidemiology of influenza. *Public Health Rep.* 1919; 34: 1823–36.

40. Ibid.

41. Sydenstricker E, King ML. Difficulties in computing civil death rates for 1918, with especial reference to epidemic influenza. *Public Health Rep.* 1920; 35: 330–45.

42. Frost WH, Sydenstricker E. Influenza in Maryland. Preliminary statistics of certain localities. *Public Health Rep.* 1919; 34:491–504.

43. Frost WH. Statistics of influenza morbidity. With special reference to certain factors in case incidence and case fatality. *Public Health Rep.* 1920; 35: 584–97.

44. Collins SD, Frost WH, Gover M, Sydenstricker E. Mortality from influenza and pneumonia in 50 large cities of the United States, 1910–1929. *Public Health Rep.* 1930; 45:2277–329.

8: Baltimore

1. WH Frost to SF Parrish, in Boston, December 27, 1937. Claude Moore Health Sciences Library, University of Virginia Health Sciences Center, Charlottesville, VA: Wade Hampton Frost Archives, Box 3, Folder 76.

2. Harvey AMcG, Brieger GH, Abrams SL, McKusick VA. *A Model of its Kind.* Vol. 1. *A Centennial History of Medicine at Johns Hopkins.* Baltimore, MD: Johns Hopkins University Press; 1989.

3. Flexner S, Flexner JT. *William Henry Welch and the Heroic Age of American Medicine.* New York, NY: Viking Press; 1941.

4. Freeman AW. *Five Million Patients: The Professional Life of a Health Officer.* New York, NY: Charles Scribner's Sons; 1946: 10.

5. Fee E. *Disease and Discovery: A History of the Johns Hopkins School of Hygiene and Public Health, 1916–1939.* Baltimore, MD: Johns Hopkins University Press; 1987.

6. WH Frost to William Welch, July 18, 1919. The original of this letter is in the Alan Mason Chesney Archives of the Medical Institutions of the Johns Hopkins University. A copy of this letter was deposited by Susan Frost Parrish at the Claude Moore Health Sciences Library, University of Virginia Health Sciences Center, Charlottesville, VA: Wade Hampton Frost Archives, Box 2, Folder 3.

7. Fee E, op. cit.

8. H Cumming to WH Frost, July 12, 1922. Claude Moore Health Sciences Library, University of Virginia Health Sciences Center, Charlottesville, VA: Wade Hampton Frost Archives, Box 3, Folder 34. WH Frost to Hugh Cumming, July 16, 1922. Claude Moore Health Sciences Library, University of Virginia Health Sciences Center, Charlottesville, VA: Wade Hampton Frost Archives, Box 9, Folder 18.

9. Fee E, op. cit: 165–66.

10. Parrish SF. Interviews conducted by Elizabeth Fee on May 5 and June 24, 1982. Transcripts deposited by Susan Frost Parrish at the Claude Moore Health Sciences Library, University of Virginia Health Sciences Center, Charlottesville, VA: Wade Hampton Frost Archives, Box 14, Folder 17.

11. Parrish SF. Undated typewritten notes. Claude Moore Health Sciences Library, University of Virginia Health Sciences Center, Charlottesville, VA: Wade Hampton Frost Archives, Box 8, Folder 20.

12. Gerczak C. Personal communication to the author.

13. Parrish SF. Undated typewritten notes. Claude Moore Health Sciences Library, University of Virginia Health Sciences Center, Charlottesville, VA: Wade Hampton Frost Archives, Box 8, Folder 12.

14. Parrish SF. Undated typewritten notes, op. cit., Box 8, Folder 20.

15. Anderson EJB. Interview by B Rutizer and SF Parrish on July 23, 1975. Tape recording of this interview deposited at the Claude Moore Health Sciences Library, University of Virginia Health Sciences Center, Charlottesville, VA: Wade Hampton Frost Archives, Box 16, Tapes 17 and 18. The recording of this interview includes many remarks and recollections by Susan Frost Parrish.

16. Ibid.

17. Ibid.

18. Parrish SF. Handwritten note dated August 25, 1984. Claude Moore Health Sciences Library, University of Virginia Health Sciences Center, Charlottesville, VA: Wade Hampton Frost Archives, Box 7, Folder 5.

19. Parrish SF. Interview conducted by E Fee on June 24, 1982. Transcript deposited by Susan Frost Parrish at the Claude Moore Health Sciences Library, University of Virginia Health Sciences Center, Charlottesville, VA: Wade Hampton Frost Archives, Box 14, Folder 17.

20. Parrish SF. Interview conducted by E Fee on May 5, 1982. Transcript deposited by Susan Frost Parrish at the Claude Moore Health Sciences Library, University of Virginia health Sciences Center, Charlottesville, VA: Wade Hampton Frost Archives, Box 14, Folder 17.

21. Ibid.

22. Parrish SF. Interview conducted by E Fee on June 24, 1982, op. cit.

23. Anderson EJB, op. cit.

24. Barton CM Jr. Interview with B Rutizer on July 23, 1975 recorded by Rutizer and deposited at the Claude Moore Health Sciences Library, University of Virginia Health Sciences Center, Charlottesville, VA: Wade Hampton Frost Archives, Box 16, Tapes 14 and 22.

25. Ibid.

26. WH Frost to SF Parrish, January 2, 1938. Claude Moore Health Sciences Library, University of Virginia Health Sciences Center, Charlottesville, VA: Wade Hampton Frost Archives, Box 3, Folder 77.

27. WH Frost to SF Parrish, December 27, 1937, op. cit.

28. Ibid.

29. Parrish SF. Interview conducted by E Fee on June 24, 1982, op. cit.

30. WH Frost to SF Parrish, November 14, (1937). Claude Moore Health Sciences Library, University of Virginia Health Sciences Center, Charlottesville, VA: Wade Hampton Frost Archives, Box 3, Folder 74.

31. Parrish SF. Handwritten notes dated November 27, 1975 and September 1984. Claude Moore Health Sciences Library, University of Virginia Health Sciences Center, Charlottesville, VA: Wade Hampton Frost Archives, Boxes 8 and 5, Folders 6 and 16.

32. Gilliam AG Jr. Personal communication to the author. Rasmussen FN. Way back when: Barely a trace of Mencken's favorite eateries. *The Baltimore Sun*, September 14, 2002. Cheslock L. *H.L. Mencken on Music: A Selection of his Writings on Music together with an Account of H.L. Mencken's Musical Life and a History of the Saturday Night Club.* New York, NY: Alfred A. Knopf; 1961

33. Barton CM Jr, op. cit.

34. Ibid.

35. Ibid.

36. Parish SF. Memorandum to B Rutizer dated July 22, 1975. Claude Moore Health Sciences Library, University of Virginia Health Sciences Center, Charlottesville, VA: Wade Hampton Frost Archives, Box 8, Folder 12. Barton CM Jr. Interview with B Rutizer on July 23, 1975 recorded by Rutizer and deposited at the Claude Moore Health Sciences Library, University of Virginia Health Sciences Center, Charlottesville, VA: Wade Hampton Frost Archives, Box 16, Tapes 14 and 22.

37. Parrish SF. Interview conducted by Elizabeth Fee on May 5, 1982, op. cit.

38. Ibid.

39. Ibid.

40. Fee E, op. cit.

41. WH Frost WH to Mr. Haxall, March 21, 1935. Claude Moore Health Sciences Library, University of Virginia Health Sciences Center, Charlottesville, VA: Wade Hampton Frost Archives, Box 3, Folder 82.

42. Parrish SF. Interview conducted by Elizabeth Fee on June 24, 1982, op. cit.

43. Ibid.

44. Anderson EJB, op. cit.

45. WH Frost to SF Parrish, July 4, (ca. 1920). Claude Moore Health Sciences Library, University of Virginia Health Sciences Center, Charlottesville, VA: Wade Hampton Frost Archives, Box 3, Folder 70.

46. Parrish SF. Remarks made during an interview with Mrs. Ivan Marty recorded by B Rutizer on July 23, 1975. Tape recording of this interview deposited at the Claude Moore Health Sciences Library, University of Virginia Health Sciences Center, Charlottesville, VA: Wade Hampton Frost Archives, Box 16, Tape 6.

47. WH Frost to SF Parrish, August 14, (1933). Claude Moore Health Sciences Library, University of Virginia Health Sciences Center, Charlottesville, VA: Wade Hampton Frost Archives, Box 3, Folder 7.

48. Parrish SF. Undated typewritten note. Claude Moore Health Sciences Library, University of Virginia Health Sciences Center, Charlottesville, VA: Wade Hampton Frost Archives, Box 8, Folder 12.

49. Parrish SF. Undated typewritten note. Claude Moore Health Sciences Library, University of Virginia Health Sciences Center, Charlottesville, VA: Wade Hampton Frost Archives, Box 12, Folder 7.

9: Professor

1. Frost WH. What every health officer should know. Epidemiology. Typescript. Address prepared for delivery before the 1937 Annual Meeting of the American Public Health Association. Claude Moore Health Sciences Library, University of Virginia Health Sciences Center, Charlottesville, VA: Wade Hampton Frost Archives, Box 4, Folder 13.

2. Frost WH. Introduction. *Snow on Cholera. Being a Reprint of Two Papers by John Snow, M.D. together with a Biographical Memoir by B.W. Richardson, M.D. and and Introduction by Wade Hampton Frost, M.D. Professor of Epidemiology, the Johns Hopkins School of Hygiene and Public Health* (Facsimile of 1936 Edition). New York, NY: Hafner Publishing Company; 1965: ix.

3. Hirsch A. *Handbook of Geographical and Historical Pathology*. London: New Sydenham Society; 1883. Cited by Frost WH. Epidemiology. In Emerson H, ed. *Nelson Loose-Leaf System: Preventive Medicine and Public Health*. Vol. 2. New York, NY: Thomas Nelson & Sons; 1928. Reprinted in Maxcy KF. *Papers of Wade Hampton Frost, M.D.: A Contribution to the Epidemiologic Method*. New York, NY: The Commonwealth Fund; 1941.

4. Frost WH. Memo dated November 8, 1919 addressed to the Committee on Organization and Activities, Johns Hopkins University, School of Hygiene and Public Health. Claude Moore Health Sciences Library, University of Virginia Health Sciences Center, Charlottesville, VA: Wade Hampton Frost Archives, Box 1, Folder 8. A copy of this memorandum is also in the Alan Chesney Mason Archives of the Medical Institutions of Johns Hopkins University, Baltimore, MD.

5. Ibid.

6. Ibid.

7. Turner TB. *Heritage of Excellence. The Johns Hopkins Medical Institutions, 1914–1947.* Baltimore, MD: The Johns Hopkins University Press; 1974.

8. Information concerning the curriculum offered in epidemiology and the department faculty is taken from appropriate numbers of the Johns Hopkins University School of Hygiene and Public Health Catalogue and Announcement, published annually the Johns Hopkins Press and bound in the Johns Hopkins Circulars available in the William W. Welch Medical Library of Johns Hopkins University.

9. Epidemiology, Etc. A Newsletter for Alumni and Friends of the Department of Epidemiology. The Johns Hopkins University School of Hygiene and Public Health. Winter 1991.

10. WH Frost to Surgeon General HS Cumming, March 14, 1921. Claude Moore Health Sciences Library, University of Virginia Health Sciences Center, Charlottesville, VA: Wade Hampton Frost Archives, Box 9, Folder 18.

11. HS Cumming, handwritten letter to WH Frost dated July 12, 1922. Claude Moore Health Sciences Library, University of Virginia Health Sciences Center, Charlottesville, VA: Wade Hampton Frost Archives, Box 3, Folder 34.

12. WH Frost to HS Cumming, July 16, 1922. Claude Moore Health Sciences Library, University of Virginia Health Sciences Center, Charlottesville, VA: Wade Hampton Frost Archives, Box 9, Folder 18.

13. Ibid.

14. WH Frost to Doctor Welch, January 3, 1926. Claude Moore Health Sciences Library, University of Virginia Health Sciences Center, Charlottesville, VA: Wade Hampton Frost Archives, Box 2, Folder 3.

15. HS Cumming H, handwritten letter addressed "Dear Frost" dated June 20, 1929. Claude Moore Health Sciences Library, University of Virginia Health Sciences Center, Charlottesville, VA: Wade Hampton Frost Archives, Box 3, Folder 35.

16. Parrish SF. Comment made during interview with Alfred Soper recorded by B Rutizer, July 27, 1975. Claude Moore Health Sciences Library, University of Virginia Health Sciences Center, Charlottesville, VA: Wade Hampton Frost Archives, Box 16, Tape 10. Details of Frost's lecture style are from the various interviews with his former students recorded by B Rutizer.

17. Wolman A. Interview recorded by B Rutizer, June 26, 1975. Claude Moore Health Sciences Library, University of Virginia Health Sciences Center, Charlottesville, VA: Wade Hampton Frost Archives, Box 16, Tape 24.

18. Stebbins E. Interview recorded by B Rutizer, July 24, 1975. Claude Moore Health Sciences Library, University of Virginia Health Sciences Center, Charlottesville, VA: Wade Hampton Frost Archives, Box 16, Tape 9.

19. Levin M. Interview recorded by B Rutizer, June 25, 1975. Claude Moore Health Sciences Library, University of Virginia Health Sciences Center, Charlottesville, VA: Wade Hampton Frost Archives, Box 16, Tape 19.

20. Wade Hampton Frost papers; Frost papers and lectures. Alan Chesney Mason Archives of the Medical Institutions of Johns Hopkins University, Baltimore, MD.

21. Ibid.

22. WH Frost to W Welch, February 10, 1930. Alan Chesney Mason Archives of the Medical Institutions of Johns Hopkins University, Baltimore, MD.

23. Vandenbrouke JP, Eelkman Rooda HM, Beukers H. Who made John Snow a hero? *Am J Epidemiology*. 1991; 133: 967–73.

24. Snow on Cholera, op. cit.

25. Ibid.

26. Panum PL. *Observations Made During the Epidemic of Measles on the Faroe Islands in the Year 1846.* New York, NY: Delta Omega Society; 1940.

27. Department of Epidemiology. Johns Hopkins Bloomberg School of Public Health. Baltimore, MD. In the departmental office is a box of uncatalogued papers related to Frost's teaching. Their provenance is unknown. Some are dated, some not. For some the author and date can be discerned or suspected with a high degree of certainty. For others the origin is more obscure.

28. Stebbins E, op. cit.

29. Levin M, op. cit.

30. Department of Epidemiology, op. cit.

31. Frost WH. Bacteriologic examination of the water supply. *Hygienic Lab Bull.* 1911; 78:73–134.

32. Wolman A, op. cit.

33. Department of Epidemiology, op. cit.

34. Merrell M. The Reed-Frost collaboration. *Am J Epidemiol.* 1976; 104:364–69.

35. Wade Hampton Frost papers, op. cit.

36. Department of Epidemiology, op. cit. Alan Chesney Mason Archives of the Medical Institutions of Johns Hopkins University, Baltimore, MD.

37. Frost WH. Some conceptions of epidemics in general. *Am J Epidemiol.* 1976; 103:141–51.

38. ReVelle CS, Lynn WR, Feldmann F. Mathematical models for the economic allocation of tuberculosis control activities in developing nations. *Am Rev Respir Dis.* 1967; 96:893–909.

39. Frost WH. Chapter 7. *Epidemiology*, op. cit.

40. Comstock GW, Bush TL, Helzlsouer, Hoffman SC. The Washington County Training Center: an exemplar of public health research in the field. *Am J Epidemiol.* 1991; 134:1023–29. Fee E. *Disease and Discovery: A History of the Johns Hopkins School of Hygiene and Public Health, 1916–1939.* Baltimore, MD: The Johns Hopkins University Press; 1987.

41. Fee E, op. cit: 182–214.

42. Draft prepared by the faculty of the Johns Hopkins School of Hygiene and Public Health dated March 1932 entitled "Proposal for Establishing a Public Health Training Area in Baltimore" and cited in Williams H. The origins of the first school of hygiene and public health and the Eastern Health District in Baltimore. *Baltimore Health News.* 1961; 38:141–52. Claude Moore Health Sciences Library, University of Virginia Health Sciences Center, Charlottesville, VA: Wade Hampton Frost Archives, Box 8, Folder 14.

43. Perkins J. Interview recorded by B Rutizer, June 27, 1975. Claude Moore Health Sciences Library, University of Virginia Health Sciences Center, Charlottesville, VA: Wade Hampton Frost Archives, Box 16, Tape 4.

44. Fee E, op. cit: 171.

45. Stebbins E, op. cit.

46. Frost WH. Correlation of sources of pollution. *Engineers and Engineering.* 1923; 15:301–304.

47. Frost WH, Streeter HW. Bacteriological studies. *Public Health Bull.* 1924; 143:184–341.

48. Chernow R. Titan. *The Life of John D. Rockefeller, Sr.* New York, NY: Random House, Inc.; 1999.

49. Ibid: 563–70.

50. Soper F. Interview recorded by B Rutizer, July 27, 1975. Claude Moore Health Sciences Library, University of Virginia Health Sciences Center, Charlottesville, VA: Wade Hampton Frost Archives, Box 16, Tape 10.

10: Epidemiologist

1. Frost WH. Introduction. *Snow on Cholera. Being a Reprint of Two Papers by John Snow, M.D. together with a Biographical Memoir by B.W. Richardson, M.D. and an Introduction by Wade Hampton Frost, M.D. Professor of Epidemiology, the Johns Hopkins School of Hygiene and Public Health* (Facsimile of 1936 Edition). New York, NY: Hafner Publishing Company; 1965: ix.

2. Stebbins E. Interview by B Rutizer recorded on June 24, 1975. Tape recording of this interview deposited at the Claude Moore Health Sciences Library, University of Virginia Health Sciences Center, Charlottesville, VA: Wade Hampton Frost Archives, Box 16, Tape 9.

3. Brailey M. Factors influencing the course of tuberculous infection in young children. *Am Rev Tuberc.* 1937; 36:347–54.

4. Frost WH, Streeter HW. Bacteriological studies. *Public Health Bull.* 1924; 143:184–341. Frost WH. A review of the work of the United States Public Health Service in investigations of stream pollution. *Public Health Rep.* 1926; 41:75–85.

5. Kinyoun C. Viability of B. typhosus in stored shell oysters. *Public Health Rep.* 1925; 40:819–23.

6. Frost WH. In Transactions of the Twenty-Third Annual Conference of State and Territorial Health Officers with the United States Public Health Service held at Washington, D.C. June 1 and 2, 1925. *Public Health Bull.* 1926; 161:89, 93–97, 108–109. Frost WH. In Transactions of the Twenty-Fourth Annual Conference of State and Territorial Health Officers with the United States Public Health Service held at Washington, D.C. May 24 and 25, 1926. *Public Health Bull.* 1927; 167: 21–23, 24. Frost WH. In Transactions of the Twenty-Fifth Annual Conference of State and Territorial Health Officers with the United States Public Health Service held at Washington, D.C. May 20 and 21, 1927. *Public Health Bull.* 1928; 178: 65–66, 68.

7. Frost WH, 1928, op. cit.

8. Frost WH. Statistics of influenza morbidity: with special reference to certain factors in case incidence and case fatality. *Public Health Rep.* 1920; 35:584–97. Reprinted in Maxcy KF. *Papers of Wade Hampton Frost, M.D.: A Contribution to the Epidemiologic Method.* New York, NY: The Commonwealth Fund; 1941: 340–58.

9. Collins SD, Frost WH, Glover M, Sydenstricker E. Mortality from influenza and pneumonia in 50 large cities of the United States, 1910–1929. *Public Health Rep.* 1930; 45: 2277–329.

10. Frost WH. Infection, immunity and disease in the epidemiology of diphtheria. With special reference to some studies in Baltimore. *J Prev Med*. 1928; 2:325–43. Reprinted in Maxcy KF, op. cit: 447–66.

11. Ibid.

12. Wheeler RE, Doull JA, Frost WH. Antitoxic immunity to diphtheria in relation to tonsillectomy. *Am J Hyg*. 1931; 14: 555–59.

13. Frost WH, Frobisher M, Jr, Van Valkenburgh VA, Levin ML. Diphtheria in Baltimore: A comparative study of morbidity, carrier prevalence and antitoxic immunity in 1921–24 and 1933–36. *Am J Hyg*. 1936; 24:568–86. Reprinted in Maxcy KF, op. cit: 467–88.

14. Frost WH, Gover M. The incidence and time distribution of common colds in several groups kept under continuous observation. *Public Health Rep*. 1932; 47:1815–41. Reprinted in Maxcy KF, op. cit: 359–92.

15. Ibid.

16. Van Valkenburgh VA, Frost WH. Acute minor respiratory diseases prevailing in a group of families residing in Baltimore, Maryland, 1928–1930: Prevalence, distribution and clinical description of observed cases. *Am J Hyg*. 1933; 17:122–53. Reprinted in Maxcy KF, op. cit: 393–426.

17. Frost WH, Van Valkenburgh VA. The minor respiratory diseases as observed during the influenza epidemic of 1928–29 and in a non-epidemic period. *Am J Hyg*. 1935; 21:647–64. Reprinted in Maxcy KF, op. cit: 427–46.

18. Frost WH. Rendering account in public health. *Am J Public Health Nations Health*. 1925; 15:394–98. Read before the Fifty-third Annual Meeting of the American Public Health Association, Detroit, MI, October 23, 1924. Reprinted in Maxcy KF, op. cit: 562–73.

19. Frost WH. Authoritative standards and association policy. *Am J Public Health Nations Health*. 1936; 26:336–42.

20. Frost WH. What every health officer should know. Epidemiology. Typescript of oral presentation. This paper was not published. Claude Moore Health Sciences Library, University of Virginia Health Sciences Center, Charlottesville, VA: Wade Hampton Frost Archives, Box 4, Folder 13.

21. Ibid.

22. Frost WH. The familial aggregation of infectious diseases. *Am J Public Health Nations Health*. 1938; 28:7–13. Reprinted in Maxcy KF, op. cit: 543–52. Quoted with permission of the American Public Health Association.

23. Panum PL. *Observations Made During the Epidemic of Measles on the Faroe Islands in the Year 1846*. New York, NY: Delta Omega Society; 1940.

24. Frost WH, 1938, op. cit.

25. Frost WH. Chapter 7. Epidemiology. Emerson H, ed. *Nelson Loose-Leaf System: Preventive Medicine and Public Health*. Vol. 2. New York: Thomas Nelson & sons; 1928. Reprinted in Maxcy KF, op. cit: 493–542. The publication date for this work was incorrectly given as 1927 by Maxcy. Later authors have made the same error, presumably having used Maxcy as their source.

26. Ibid.

27. Merrell M. The Reed-Frost collaboration. *Am J Epidemiol*. 1976; 104: 364–69.

28. Frost WH. Some conceptions of epidemics in general. *Am J Epidemiol*. 1976; 103:141–51.

29. Department of Commerce. Bureau of the Census. Mortality Statistics 1920. Twenty-First Annual Report. Washington, DC: Government Printing Office, 1923. Department of Commerce. Bureau of the Census. Mortality Statistics 1930. Thirty-First Annual Report. Washington, DC: Government Printing Office; 1934.

30. Centers for Disease Control and Prevention. Reported Tuberculosis in the United States, 2001. Atlanta, GA: United States Department of health and Human Services; 2002.

31. Gerczak C. Department of Epidemiology, Johns Hopkins Bloomberg School of Public Health. Ms. Gerczak has studied the life of Miriam Brailey and kindly shared much of her information with the author.

32. Brailey M. Factors influencing the course of tuberculous infection in young children. *Am Rev Tuberc.* 1937; 36:347–54. For more comprehensive studies from the Harriet Lane Clinic, see Brailey M. A study of tuberculous infection and mortality in the children of tuberculous households. *Am J Hyg.* 1940; 31(Sec. A):1–43 and Brailey ME. *Tuberculosis in White and Negro Children.* Vol. 2. *The Epidemiologic Aspects of the Harriet Lane Study.* Cambridge, MA: Harvard University Press; 1958.

33. Brailey M, 1937, op. cit.

34. Zeidberg LD, Gass RS, Dillon A, Hutcheson RH. The Williamson County tuberculosis study: a twenty-four-year epidemiologic study. *Am Rev Respir Dis.* 1963; 87(Suppl):1–88.

35. EL Bishop to Mrs. WH Frost, May 19, 1949. Claude Moore Health Sciences Library, University of Virginia Health Sciences Center, Charlottesville, VA: Wade Hampton Frost Archives, Box 3, Folder 7.

36. Frost WH. Risk of persons in familial contact with pulmonary tuberculosis. *Am J Public Health Nations Health.* 1933; 23:426–32. Reprinted in Maxcy KF, op. cit: 582–92.

37. Ibid.

38. Zeidberg LD, Gass RS, Dillon A, Hutcheson RH, op. cit.

39. Puffer RR, Doull JA, Gass RS, Murphy WJ, Williams WC. Use of the index case in the study of tuberculosis in Williamson County. *Am J Public Health.* 1942; 32:601–605.

40. Frost WH, 1933, op. cit.

41. Zeidberg LD, Gass RS, Dillon A, Hutcheson RH, op. cit.

42. Comstock GW. Interview with the author, October 2, 2002.

43. Comstock GW. Early studies of tuberculosis. In Garfinkel L, Ochs O, Mushinski M, eds. *Selection, Follow-up, and Analysis in Prospective Studies: A Workshop. Proceedings of a Conference Held at the Waldorf-Astoria Hotel, New York, N.Y. October 3–5, 1983.* National Cancer Institute Monograph Number 67; 1985: 23–27.

44. Zeidberg LD, Gass RS, Dillon A, Hutcheson RH, op. cit.

45. Zeidberg LD, Dillon A, Gass RS. Risk of developing tuberculosis among children of tuberculous parents. *Am Rev Tuberc.* 1954; 70:1008–19.

46. Puffer RR, Stewart HC, Gass RS. Tuberculosis in household associates: the influence of age and relationship. *Am Rev Tuberc.* 1945; 52:89–103.

47. Puffer RR, Gass RS, Murphy WJ, Williams WC. Tuberculosis studies in Tennessee: prevalence of tuberculous infection and disease in white and colored families as revealed at the time of investigation. *Am J Hyg.* 1941; 34:71–78.

48. Daniel TM, Baum GL. *Drama and Discovery: The Story of Histoplasmosis*. Westport, CT: Greenwood Press; 2002.

49. Frost WH. The outlook for the eradication of tuberculosis. *Am Rev Tuberc*. 1935; 32:644–50.

50. Frost WH. How much control of tuberculosis? *Am J Public Health Nations Health*. 1937; 27:759–66. Reprinted in Maxcy KF, op. cit: 601–12.

51. Frost WH. The age selection of mortality from tuberculosis in successive decades. *Am J Hyg*. 1939; 30:91–96. Reprinted in Frost WH. The age selection of mortality from tuberculosis in successive decades. *Am J Epidemiol*. 1995; 141:91–96. Reprinted in Maxcy KF, op. cit: 593–600.

52. Ibid. For further discussion of this concept, see also Daniel TM. *Pioneers of Medicine and Their Impact on Tuberculosis*. Rochester, NY: University of Rochester Press; 2000: 173–77.

53. Comstock GW. Invited commentary of "The Age Selection of Mortality from Tuberculosis in Successive Decades." *Am J Epidemiol*. 1995; 141:3.

54. Andvord KF. What can we learn by following the development of tuberculosis from one generation to another? *Int J Tuberc Lung Dis*. 2002; 6:562–68. This reference is to a translation in English originally made by Gerard Wijsmulller at the request of George Comstock. For commentary on this paper, see Blomberg B, Rieder HL, Enarson DA. Kristian Andvord's impact on the understanding of tuberculosis epidemiology. *Int J Tuberc Lung Dis*. 2002; 6:557–59.

55. Wade Hampton Frost papers. Alan Chesney Mason Archives of the Medical Institutions of Johns Hopkins University, Baltimore, MD.

56. Perkins J. Interview recorded by B Rutizer on June 27, 1975. Claude Moore Health Sciences Library, University of Virginia Health Sciences Center, Charlottesville, VA: Wade Hampton Frost Archives, Box 16, Tape 4.

57. Metchnikoff E, Burnet E, Tarassevitch L. Recherches sur l'épidémiologie de la tuberculose dans les steppes des Kalmouks. *Ann Inst Pasteur*. 1911; 25:785–804.

58. Frost WH, 1939, op cit.

59. Ibid.

60. Comstock GW, op. cit.

11: Sunset and Evening Star

1. WH Frost, unfinished hand-written letter to his brother, Thomas Frost, dated March 15th [1923]. Thomas Frost died the following day. Claude Moore Health Sciences Library, University of Virginia Health Sciences Center, Charlottesville, VA: Wade Hampton Frost Archives, Box 3, Folder 89.

2. WH Frost to SH Frost. Johns Hopkins University, School of Hygiene and Public Health. Claude Moore Health Sciences Library, University of Virginia Health Sciences Center, Charlottesville, VA: Wade Hampton Frost Archives, Box 4, Folder 49.

3. Owens J. Wade Hampton Frost. Obituary editorial. *The [Baltimore] Sun*. May 3, 1938.

4. Wade Hampton Frost. Obituary editorial. *Am J Public Health Nations Health.* 1938; 28:733–34.

5. Transcript provided by Charlotte Gerczak, Department of Epidemiology, Johns Hopkins Bloomberg School of Public Health. Quoted with permission.

6. Sedgwick Memorial Medal awarded to Wade Hampton Frost, M.D. *Am J Public Health Nations Health.* 1938; 28:1357–58.

Index